Stroke

A Practical Guide For New Patients And Their Caregivers

Stroke

A Practical Guide For New Patients And Their Caregivers

Mark Knoblauch PhD

Kiremma Press
Houston, TX

Printed in the United States of America

Disclaimer: The information provided within this book is for general informational purposes only. While we try to keep the information up-to-date and correct, there are no representations or warranties, express or implied, about the completeness, accuracy, reliability, suitability or availability with respect to the information contained in this book for any purpose. Any use of this information is at your own risk.

This book is not intended as a substitute for the medical advice of licensed medical providers. The reader should regularly consult with their physician in matters relating to his/her health and particularly with respect to any symptoms that may require diagnosis or medical attention

www.authorMK.com

ISBN: 978-1-7333210-4-4

To my mom – whose own affliction made me realize just how much I have taken for granted

Table of Contents

Introduction...xi

Chapter 1: The Brain..21

Chapter 2 – Stroke 49

Chapter 3 – Risk Factors for Stroke 69

Chapter 4 – Stroke Mimics 87

Chapter 5 – Diagnosing Stroke 95

Chapter 6 – The stroke care team..................117

Chapter 7 – Stroke management....................127

Chapter 8 – Stroke rehabilitation...................135

Chapter 9 – Reducing Future Stroke Risk......167

Chapter 10 – Caregivers 173

Conclusion 193

Introduction

You've had a stroke. It's a phrase that ranks alongside the most serious of medical conditions a patient can experience. Instantly, the patient and his or her loved ones, friends, and even coworkers are forced to understand a whole new person who may hold little resemblance to the person they knew previously. Gone are the witty personality and poised responses, replaced in many cases with confused looks and slow, strained movements. Perhaps worst of all is that it strikes with no warning – no allowance of time to prepare for this major upheaval that affects so many aspects of life. Instead of a slow onset of symptoms over time, the first indication of stroke may be a complete loss of speech or memory, or the inability to recognize even the closest of family members. Unlike so many other medical conditions that allow the patient to start treatments in an attempt to ward off the ailment, stroke patients and those around them are often thrust sight-unseen into damage-control mode, trying frantically to identify the extent of brain impairment while simultaneously seeking to grasp the magnitude of what has happened to them or their loved one.

For some patients, the consequences of stroke are short-lived as they soon make significant strides in getting back to their prior self. Their memory improves, speech becomes more easily understood, and they are soon able to walk unsupported again. Within a few months they might even be back to how they were prior to the stroke. Other patients, though, may not be as fortunate. Those who suffer severe stroke may never return to their prior self, instantly and permanently entering into a life which they have little to no control over. Such becomes the life of a stroke patient.

For me, my introduction to the personal side of stroke came on a chilly fall evening. As much as anyone might say they remember where they were when they heard President Kennedy was shot, or when they learned about the 9/11 attacks, I clearly remember pressing the button on my truck's touchscreen to answer the incoming phone call from my brother. I expected nothing more than a typical conversation, thinking he might ask for some assistance with a friend's job application or tell me about one of his kids' accomplishments. My suspicions were so low that I didn't even prep him that my 10-year-old daughter was seated next to me in the truck, as it had been so long since I'd had any kind of consequential phone call with him that I gave myself no reason to suspect anything more than another innocent conversation.

"Hey", came his response to my phone greeting.
"Yes, sir!", I replied.
"Mom just had a stroke".
"WHAT?!?!?"

I had heard him clearly, but the shock of the news elicited a response from my mouth before my brain could fully process the message. I glanced over at my daughter, who at that moment had the look on her face that meant tears were soon to follow. My next thoughts turned to aggravation at myself for not taking the call privately to avoid the drama soon to arrive from a 10-year-old who now knows something bad has happened to her nana. Thoughts of *what will this do to my daughter* and *how do I talk to her about what a stroke is* raced through my mind, but I instantly snapped back to the fact that I don't have any real information about the situation and needed more.

The next few minutes were filled with a dizzying back and forth with my brother about the sketchy details of the situation. I was certainly hearing the limited information he was relaying, but processing it all was quite problematic as I was being bombarded with flashbacks to childhood memories with my mom and wondering how and why something like this could happen to her. At the same time my mind was trying to mentally compute a travel itinerary that would allow me the most efficient way to get up to see her, which in turn required some mental calculus in trying to synchronize upcoming sports and school schedules for our kids, existing work responsibilities for myself and my wife, and wondering what to pack for a trip of unknown duration. All of this was rushing through my mind despite the fact that we still had only fragmented information about her condition and without me realizing that I'm probably in a mild state of shock.

While everyone's introduction to the world of stroke is unique to them, chances are high that every person who learns of a close friend or loved one's stroke can identify some similarity to what I experienced in those initial minutes. Stroke is well known for its detrimental effects on the patient, but it can also create quite the psychological wallop to the patient's family and friends. In an instant, life's normal pace can be upended by a debilitating and devastating medical condition that arrived as unexpectedly as it was unwelcomed.

A small advantage I had in this situation was that I have been employed in healthcare, which allowed me to mentally organize some pertinent issues such as risk factors and brain function. I've even spent years teaching at the collegiate level about medical conditions including stroke. I quickly learned, however, that when something as severe as stroke happens to someone close to you, it still manages to catch you off-guard. As I spent time with my mom in her neuro-intensive care room, I began reading up on stroke in order to strengthen my own knowledge foundation as to stroke's causes, effects, and expected outcomes. I found myself scanning through material from a variety of sources ranging from blogs to journal articles to online medical textbooks. Each had its own benefit, whether it be the newest updates to published stroke management guidelines, a patient's beautifully written insight into their own experience with stroke, or the latest research into a highly-technical treatment. As I dug further in my own reading, I began to suspect that there are likely a *lot* of stroke patients and caregivers who are also seeking information related to stroke but don't have access to – or aren't aware of – the array of quality medical information that exists on stroke. These same individuals would likely benefit from a single source that summarizes the latest medical research without all the intense medical terminology.

That thought process – specifically, compiling the available stroke research – ultimately served as the stimulus for putting together this book. I have always loved writing and spent years as a scientist navigating and even producing my own medical research, and thought that writing a book about stroke would be a worthwhile project. Soon after, I started poring through books, websites, blogs, and many medical journals. But as I started collecting the information, I quickly learned that the seriousness and frequency of stroke has resulted in a *lot* of information existing about stroke – so much so that the amount of available information quickly became overwhelming. I found stroke articles in major medical journals but also learned that there are journals dedicated just to a specific area of stroke such as rehabilitation which may publish 30 or more articles in their specialty *every month.* In reading source after source, it was easy to find evidence which supported prior research as often as

I found evidence that *contradicted* prior reports. Over time, this vast amount of information required me to start thinking more about 'what not to include' than my original plan of 'what to include' as I realized the scope of just how much information on stroke existed. If I sat back and thought about it long enough I found that it could become quite daunting at times – such as when having to decide whether to include information about one new study that contradicted ten existing studies, or trying to determine what level of detail to go into regarding the physiologic mechanisms of anti-coagulant therapy.

The end result of that seemingly formidable process is this book – a book written for stroke patients and their caregivers with the goal of helping them understand stroke. To accomplish this objective, the book approaches stroke initially from a foundational level before moving into particular aspects of stroke. First we will take a look at the brain, outlining its main functions including which areas of the brain are responsible for regulating movement, personality, etc. Because blood flow and circulation are a key aspect of stroke, we will also discuss blood flow within the brain, including oxygen's role in brain metabolism. In the next chapter we will focus on stroke itself, discussing the types of stroke that can occur as well as their primary causes. We will then outline some of the statistics of stroke specific to how often they occur, who is affected, and various data regarding each stroke type. This is followed by a chapter discussing the various risk factors inherent to both initial and recurrent stroke, highlighting those factors which can help reduce one's risk of suffering a subsequent stroke.

The middle chapters of the book will focus on events surrounding the diagnosis and immediate care of stroke. Whereas an initial part of stroke care is spent trying to recognize that a stroke has occurred, we will first discuss stroke 'mimics' which are those medical conditions that closely resemble stroke. Then, because you likely witnessed much of the medical care provided in the hours and days after stroke, we will outline some of the procedures, technology, and processes used in diagnosing stroke which can help you to understand the many tests and measures you may have observed taking place during the diagnostic process. Then, because stroke care itself involves what seems to be a revolving team of healthcare professionals, we will spend a chapter describing the many team members regarding their level of training and their primary responsibilities.

Finally, we will turn our focus towards the recovery phase of stroke. First, we'll spend a chapter discussing the steps used in managing stroke in the immediate hours after diagnosis, followed by a chapter outlining the major concepts and principles associated with stroke rehabilitation that patients are exposed to on the road to stroke recovery. Finally, we will devote a chapter to stroke caretakers who are responsible for providing care after the patient leaves the hospital. Although the patient is rightfully the center of focus when it comes to stroke care, research has revealed key information about caretakers in terms of the role they serve and the challenges they face, and we will outline some of that important information.

Whereas stroke is no doubt an unexpected yet major event in an individual's life and the lives of those around them, this book is designed to help you as a stroke patient or caregiver navigate the long journey on the way to recovery – whatever level of recovery that may be. To do this, I have worked to make this book as informative and factual as possible, with the majority of information taken directly from the medical literature. I have also included citations within the text so that if you are interested in learning more about the information you are reading, you will have at your disposal a list of references outlining where you can find additional information on that particular topic.

In closing, it must be made clear that this book is not in any way intended to guide your stroke care or suggest what kind of care should be provided. Those types of decisions should always be made by the medical professionals directly involved in you or your loved one's stroke care and are dependent upon a wealth of factors that are specific to the stroke patient. Rather, this book is intended to be an educational source for you, written to inform you of the processes and events surrounding stroke and stroke care. It is my hope that this book brings you a better understanding of stroke itself, and allows you to have meaningful and productive conversations with those healthcare providers involved. With that being said, let's set out on our journey towards a better understanding of stroke.

Chapter 1: The Brain

In mapping out the chapters for this book, it didn't take me long to realize that there were a variety of paths down which this book could go. As I started compiling the major concepts I wanted to cover – which eventually became individual chapters – I focused on areas that mirrored my own interests when learning as much as I could about stroke. I knew that I wanted to include topics such as the signs and symptoms of stroke as well as rehabilitation, but I also wanted to be able to outline what a stroke is so that patients and caregivers have access to the foundational concepts inherent to stroke. Doing that – explaining what a stroke is – created a bit of turmoil in my own mind. On the one hand, I could start elaborating on the physiology of stroke and how it affects the brain. But on the other hand, I started to feel that the book wouldn't be complete if I jumped immediately into a discussion of how a stroke affects the brain without first providing you the reader a bit of an overview of the brain itself.

Therefore, this first chapter aims to provide you some basic fundamental information about the brain and how it functions. This will then allow us to later have a more focused discussion about how stroke impacts the brain. My intent is to not get so detailed in brain function that this chapter resembles an anatomy course review. Instead, I want the chapter to introduce you to the brain's basic anatomy and function as each relates to stroke so that we can later learn how the brain is affected by stroke. This will allow us in the next chapter to better understand concepts such as why stroke affects everyone differently as well as how and why daily life can be so severely impacted by stroke.

The Brain

The brain is an incredibly complex organ and is involved to some degree in pretty much everything we do. Researchers have analyzed and studied the brain for years, and while much progress in our understanding of the brain has been made, there are still many, many characteristics that we don't yet understand. Still, as amazingly beautiful as the brain can be in giving us our ability to have thoughts, and memories, and experiences in life, it is also inherently fragile. Even a seemingly simple hit to the head can for some individuals cause life-changing alterations and remove any resemblance to the person we once knew. Yet at other times the brain shows an amazing resistance to injury and can allow a person to walk away unharmed from what was feared to be life-altering trauma. These opposing outcomes reflect how a number of individual factors play a role in whether a loss of brain function may occur in response to injury or illness – factors such as the degree of trauma absorbed by the brain, immune system integrity, age, fitness level, co-existing conditions, medical history, and so on. Because of these factors, brain injuries such as stroke can differ immensely across affected individuals.

In terms of its composition, the brain itself is a collection of nerves. Best-guess estimates suggest that there are approximately 100 billion neurons in the brain, each of which has around 7,000 connections with other neurons[1]. This results in approximately one quadrillion (i.e. one thousand trillion, or 10^{15}) interconnections within our brain. It is these interconnections that make us who we are – our personality, our beliefs, our memories, and all the other wonderful and amazing concepts inherent to the brain which we still know so little about.

When it comes to the brain and this network of trillions of interconnections, there is something called the 'Principle of Sufficient Reason' which can loosely apply to the importance of this vast network. This principle, attributed to Gottfried Wilhelm, outlines that everything that exists has an explanation for its existence[2]. Therefore, if something doesn't serve a viable purpose, nature gets rid of it. In other words, if nature at some distant point in the past decided that we as humans require 1 quadrillion neural connections to function normally, then every single connection must have some role and thereby has importance. Suddenly remove or disrupt a few of those connections and some degree of consequence will result, even if we never consciously know that the consequence occurs. For example, a noticeable outcome from the death of ten neurons within the brain will likely never be recognized, depending on the task assigned to those neurons. Perhaps we take a microsecond longer to think of a particular word, or we lose the ability to access some faint and distant memory as a result, but most likely the consequence will go unnoticed.

In situations where a greater degree of neural damage occurs, the affected individual tends to reveal the inherent damage through a noticeable loss of some characteristic body function. This loss of function may occur through an alteration in balance, memory, or speech, and result in what others around him or her recognize as the signs of stroke. Unfortunately, although the effects of this damage may be evident to others, the individual himself or herself may be oblivious to the loss. This can occur in situations where the very neurons responsible for an individual's self-recognition of body function are themselves damaged – something we will discuss shortly. In other words, an individual can't determine something is wrong if the portion of the brain that provides an individual the ability to recognize 'normal' from 'not normal' is itself compromised. To understand this concept a little better, let's delve into an overview of how the brain functions.

The Neuron

Just as all organs of the body are comprised of cells, the brain is comprised of many billions of specialized cells known as neurons. Despite being closely packed together, nerves of the brain operate independently yet also cluster into groups to coordinate functions such as hearing, vision, breathing, recording memories, and any other number of body functions

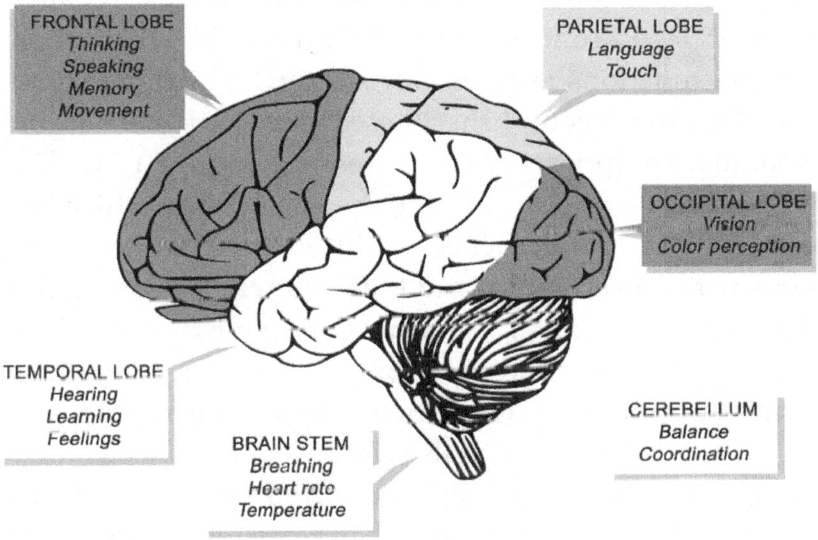

Figure 1.1. The brain consists of neurons which are organized into areas known as lobes, each specializing in the coordination of specific body functions

required for us to be 'normal'. So while the average person might see the brain as one large grayish mass, a neurologist would direct his or her attention to the section responsible for the processing of hearing, or the area that controls arm and hand movement, or the lobe which allows you rational thoughts (see Figure 1.1). As long as the connections for those areas remain stable, there should be no real disruptions to normal function.

The thousands of interconnections each neuron has with other neurons serves to create the 'network' our brain uses to perform its vast array of functions. The neuron is designed to perform a variety of tasks such as receiving sensory input (e.g. sensation, heat, pressure, etc.) from our external world, sending signals to cause our muscles to contract, and coordinating the regulation of body functions required for survival. To understand how a neuron accomplishes these tasks, think of a neuron as similar in appearance to a tree (see Figure 1.2). The neuron has three primary sections – dendrites, which are analogous to tree branches, a cell body called the soma (similar to a tree trunk), and the axon with its associated terminals (tree roots). Dendrites are the neuron's input receptors and are used to receive information from other neurons to which it is connected. The soma is responsible for processing those signals within its cell nucleus, and the axons send out signals as directed by the soma. In essence, a neuron is its own little processing organ which can receive input, make a decision based upon that input, and send out a response to that input. Multiply that ability by the trillions of interconnections organized and coordinated within the brain, and you can start to comprehend the neural foundation that establishes our individual personalities, tastes, and dislikes as humans.

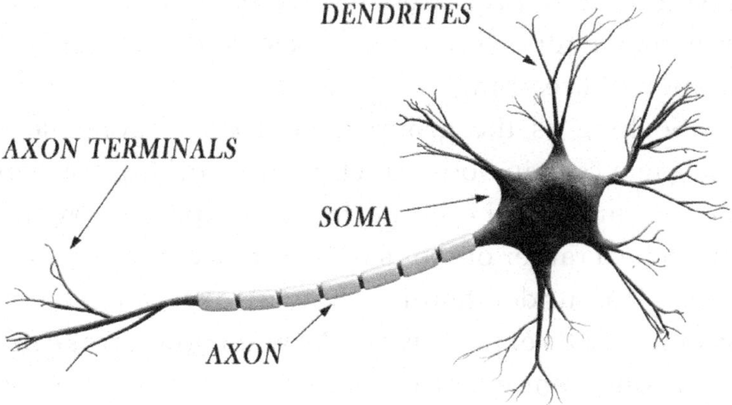

Figure 1.2. The neuron consists of sections responsible for receiving input (dendrites), processing that input (soma), and sending signals through its terminals

Brain organization

Now that we have outlined the basics of the neuron, we can begin to recognize how neurons within the brain work together to perform particular functions. As discussed, the brain is not one singular mass that performs a specific function. Rather, the brain is multi-functional in nature based on its individual sections. Some areas of the brain focus on motor function that is responsible for producing and controlling physical movements such as leg extension or helping to maintain one's balance. Other distinct regions of the brain regulate sensations such as touch or heat, while other areas are in charge of psychological aspects such as attention or aggressiveness. Some sections of the brain are even involved in body processes that we have no real control over as they happen on a subconscious level, such as the regulation of breathing.

So long as the grouped neurons responsible for regulating a certain body function are working correctly, that body function should perform as expected. While it seems to be a rather obvious notion, this concept remains the basis for understanding how stroke can affect an individual. Let's explain why. As you know, stroke itself is not a consistent event in that not everyone who has a stroke suffers the same effects. This is not necessarily true for conditions such as the common cold, as cold sufferers can generally expect relatively similar symptoms including runny nose, dry cough, and sore throat. The source of these cold symptoms is a virus which attacks the body and causes a disruption to the body's normal processes, resulting in what we see as the traditional common cold. The basis for stroke, however, is a bit different. Although stroke, like the common cold, has a consistent cause – in stroke's case it is blockage of blood flow to the brain – the location of that blockage dictates the patient's signs and symptoms. Because different areas of the brain control different body functions, the effects of stroke are ultimately dependent upon the location of the blockage.

It's interesting to note that much of our early understanding of the brain's separate regions exists due to these various effects of stroke. In the early days of brain research, a stroke patient's loss of a body function(s) was plotted against the area of the brain known to have experienced blood flow disruption[3]. Over time, researchers were able to detail out the various regions of the brain and identify the primary functional responsibilities of those regions. This process happens often in medicine, as the occurrence or even repeated occurrence of a disease like stroke allows us to learn more about the disease itself. With each unfortunate event, we hopefully learn something we did not previously know, in turn contributing to our overall knowledge base. Next, we will take a deeper look at the various areas of the brain to see how the organization of neurons coordinates particular body functions.

Regions

One classification system used in detailing the various areas of the brain is to separate the brain into regions. There are three primary regions generally recognized, each unique and functionally separate from each other. As we will see, however, although each region has specific assigned roles, these roles may be shared between regions in order to facilitate normal body function.

Forebrain

The forebrain is the largest region of the brain and contains the visible cerebral cortex as well as a number of other deeper structures including the thalamus, hypothalamus, and pituitary gland (see Figure 1.3). Together, the structures of the forebrain make up approximately two-thirds of the brain's total mass. Structurally, the forebrain consists of separate left and right hemispheres, and these hemispheres are connected to each other by a large network of nerves called the *corpus callosum*.

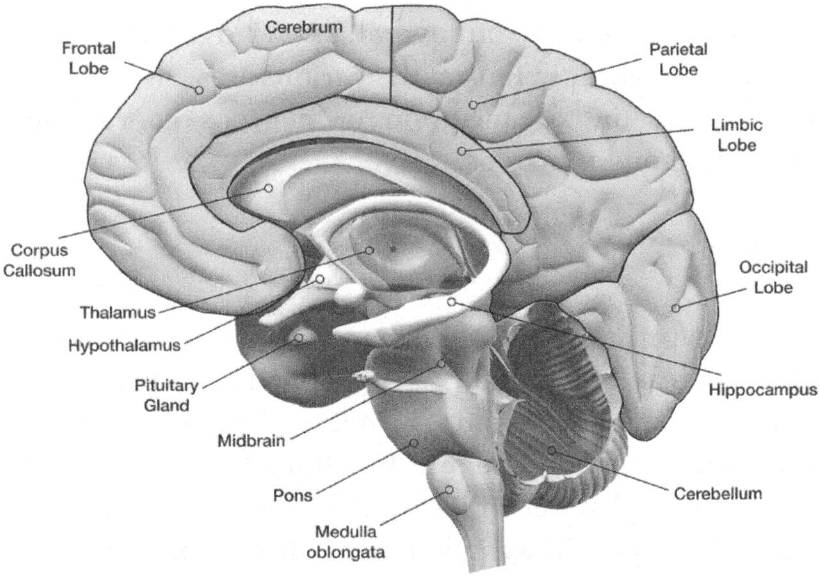

Figure 1.3. Within the interior of the brain are a variety of structures that are each responsible for controlling certain functions within the body

Because of the design of the forebrain, many neural commands from one side of the body cross to the opposite side of the brain through the corpus callosum. This results in the right hemisphere primarily controlling functions on the left side of the body while the left hemisphere oversees functions on the right side of the body. Through this design, stroke-associated complications that are evident on the right side of the body may indicate damage to the left side of the brain. Along with being separated into these left and right hemispheres, the forebrain is often further classified into *lobes* which have more defined roles, as we will discuss shortly.

Midbrain

Deep inside the lower portion of the brain is a small area known as the *midbrain*. Despite its relatively small size in comparison to the other two regions, the midbrain regulates vital functions including some involvement in the processing of vision and hearing stimuli, aiding in muscle movement, regulation of pain, and even plays a role in sleep and overall alertness[4,5]. The midbrain also has an important role in coordinating certain reflexes such as those involved with pupil changes in response to dark or light[6].

Hindbrain

You have likely heard of a portion of the brain referred to as the 'brain stem'. If so, what is being described are both the midbrain and hindbrain areas of the brain which together comprise the brain stem. As an individual unit, the hindbrain consists of the spinal cord, cerebellum, and those portions of the brain stem not represented by the midbrain. The hindbrain is considered to be the 'oldest' portion of our brain in the evolutionary process[7] and has important roles in survival-related functions such as those involved in heart rate and breathing, balance and coordination, muscle function, and coordinating reflexes, among many other responsibilities[8]. Interestingly, the cerebellum, a walnut-shaped structure on the backside of the brain, has recently been suggested to play a more intricate role in many of the body's functions than previously thought[9], and despite making up only around 10% of brain mass, the cerebellum contains 80% of all the brain's neurons![10].

Lobes

You are probably somewhat familiar with the various sections of the brain commonly known as 'lobes' (see figure 1.1). When you see an image of the brain you are generally looking at the aforementioned forebrain which is itself further divided into four lobes known as the frontal, parietal, temporal, and occipital lobes. Each lobe is responsible for coordinating a unique set of responsibilities, yet like the various regions of the brain there exists some shared responsibilities between lobes.

Frontal lobe

The frontal lobe can be found on the most forward part of the brain and extends back to a structure known as the 'central sulcus', a deep fold in the top area of the brain[11]. The frontal lobe is largely responsible for much of our cognitive reasoning (i.e. our ability to take information and analyze it), emotions, language, and voluntary muscle movements[11].

Within the frontal lobe are specialized areas of neurons responsible for coordinating specific functions. For example, the motor cortex of the frontal lobe has a role in helping us prepare and coordinate our physical movement. The prefrontal cortex regulates what is known as 'high-level cognitive functioning' and is responsible for management of our 'thinking'-type skills such as the understanding of concepts, decision making, critical thinking, brainstorming (including creativity), or understanding rules. The frontal lobe also contains a specialized section known as Broca's area which guides our language production through an intricate synchronization of our breathing and mouth movements during speech.

Parietal lobe

The parietal lobe is located just behind the frontal lobe and is involved in the processing of information derived from the body's various senses (e.g. sight, touch, sound, etc.). The parietal lobe also processes sensory input from our feet, joints, and other touch-related areas as required for spatial awareness that allows us to recognize our body's position within our surroundings[12]. For example, knowing how far to bend your leg in order to step up onto a flight of stairs requires self-awareness of how much your knee is bent and how high your foot is raised off of the floor. The parietal lobe helps coordinate those movements without requiring you to physically look down to check. Your parietal lobe also plays a role in our understanding of the relationship between numbers, distance, and counting, and it helps coordinate our attention span, among other duties[13].

Occipital lobe

In the back of the brain is the smallest of the four lobes – the occipital lobe. This lobe is responsible for interpreting input received from our eyes. This input can be summarized as 'vision' but is actually made up of multiple aspects of vision such as the recognition of color and shape as well as the processing of motion that is picked up by our eyes[14]. Because we have two eyes, the occipital lobe is able to coordinate those separate images into one image that provides us our depth perception. Additionally, the occipital lobe interacts with the temporal lobe to provide our facial recognition capability as well as some aspects of memory, along with other roles[15, 16].

Temporal lobe

The fourth and final lobe of the brain is the temporal lobe, located on the lower sides of the forebrain. The temporal lobe's primary responsibilities center around the processing of memories, auditory input, and emotions[17]. Specific to auditory processing, for example, the temporal lobe is responsible for us being able to focus on one conversation in a loud room (i.e. 'selective hearing'). The temporal lobe also has a degree of influence on visual processing such as object recognition and is involved in our ability to comprehend and understand language.

Blood flow in the brain

Now that we've discussed the neuron and how neurons are grouped together in particular areas of the brain, let's turn our attention to another area involved in stroke – blood flow. The uninterrupted delivery of blood to the brain is critical for the neuron to function normally, and any disruption to blood flow can halt the delivery of oxygen to the neuron. If oxygen cannot be accessed by the neuron for a long enough time, the neuron dies. If enough neurons die, the brain can lose a portion of its processing ability, depending upon where the damage occurred. As we have just discussed, a variety of specialized areas exist within the brain; therefore, we can now start to understand how the debilitating effects of stroke are dependent upon where in the brain the blood flow was disrupted. In this next section we will look at how blood flow and its critical oxygen passenger are delivered to the brain. In addition, we will discuss blood vessel anatomy in order to better understand the underlying processes involved with stroke.

Oxygen Demand

Like all cells in our body, neurons require oxygen to function. To deliver an adequate supply of oxygen, blood vessels serve as a pathway to allow blood from the heart to reach all cells of the body. Heart rate, in conjunction with breathing rate, is coordinated to the level of oxygen needed by the cells. If our body needs an increased level of oxygen – such as might occur after we run up a flight of stairs – our heart and breathing rates increase in order to meet the heightened oxygen demand of cells involved in allowing us to run up those stairs. Conversely, during periods of rest our oxygen demand is at its lowest. This corresponds to when our body exhibits its slowest heart and breathing rates.

Depriving the body of oxygen has two unique but very different consequences depending on the amount of time involved. You've performed one of these methods hundreds of times by simply holding your breath. Holding your breath does, by definition, deprive the body of its required continuous supply of oxygen, but there is little real danger in doing so because the period without oxygen is so short in nature. As the oxygen already in your blood continues to get used up and the carbon dioxide levels increase, your body signals the brain to inhale. If you continue to hold your breath, you enter a stage of *hypoxia* as you are starting to starve your body of oxygen. Hold your breath long enough and you will simply fall unconscious. At that point, neurons within your hindbrain go into action and cause you to immediately start breathing again despite being unconscious.

The second method of depriving oxygen to the body has more significant consequences as it deals with long-term deprivation of oxygen to the body's cells. Such an event would occur when blood flow to a cell is disrupted due to the vessel being damaged from an incision, or if a person stops breathing even when unconscious. All cells need oxygen, but cell types have different oxygen demands. If, for example, you receive an incision on your finger there will indeed be a disruption of blood flow to some number of cells in the area of that cut; however, as we will discuss shortly, cells in certain areas of the body are quite resilient to a change in blood flow and will typically be able to survive long enough for the incision to clot and blood flow to slowly be restored over time.

Neurons of the brain are of a bit more concern when it comes to blood flow than what might occur in a cut on your finger. Neurons have a very high oxygen demand, requiring about 20% of all inhaled oxygen[18]. When acting out the aforementioned holding of one's breath, neurons have access to the bloodstream which still contains some degree of oxygen within its red blood cells. So for the minute or two you can hold your breath, neurons will be fine. If, however, blood flow to the neuron is cut off due to vessel damage or blockage, or if blood flow no longer occurs due to events such as a heart attack, oxygenated blood can no longer reach the neuron. When this occurs for a long enough time, the neuron – like all of the body's cells – will eventually die.

As mentioned, cell types are not all built the same when it comes to oxygen need. For example, cell types such as neurons have a critical need for oxygen and can begin to die after just a few minutes without oxygen[18] while fingers and toes experiencing amputation can successfully be reattached six or more hours later (though possibly with some degree of functional loss such as diminished sensation). This indicates that the cell types within our fingers and toes are much less sensitive to oxygen deprivation than neurons. In fact, as outlined in the following table, neurons are the most sensitive cells in our body when it comes to oxygen demand.

Table 1.1. Time to reach tissue hypoxia[19]

Tissue	Survival time
Brain	<3 min
Kidney and liver	15-20 min
Skeletal muscle	60-90 min
Vascular smooth muscle	24-72 h
Hair and nails	Several days

Blood pathways

The heart is responsible for pushing oxygenated blood through the various blood vessel types known as arteries, capillaries, and veins (see Figure 1.4). Each

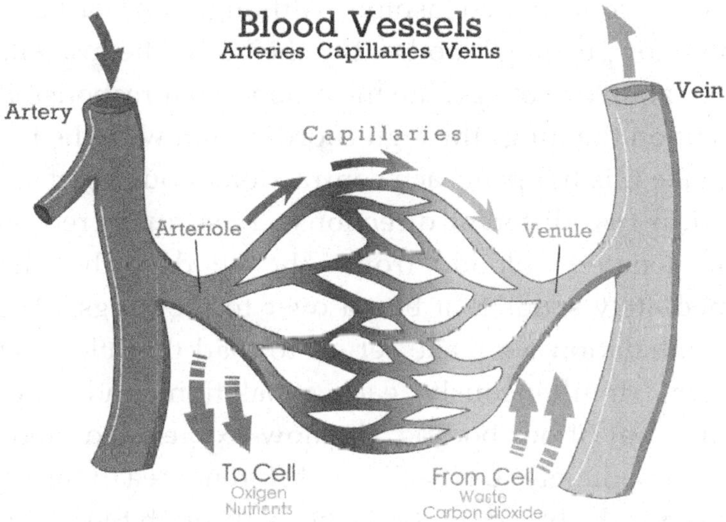

Figure 1.4. Blood leaves the heart through arteries which eventually turn into arterioles and then capillaries. Once oxygen exchange has occurred with the cells, the blood passes through venules before being returned to the heart through veins.

vessel has a specific role in delivering blood throughout the body including the brain. Arteries carry oxygenated blood from the heart out toward the body's cells. As the arteries become smaller, they transition into arterioles before ultimately becoming capillaries, the vessel type where oxygen exchange occurs with individual cells. Once the oxygen has been delivered to the cells, the capillary begins to transition back into larger vessels, first becoming a venule before eventually becoming the veins which carry the now-unoxygenated blood back to the heart.

In order for the heart to push *oxygenated* blood throughout the body there are two systems that must work in a coordinated fashion. Although the heart is well known for pushing blood out to the body, the heart itself has no ability to oxygenate the blood. That responsibility falls upon the lungs through coordination with the heart. To make this happen, each contraction of our heart sends blood in two different directions. First, upon receiving unoxygenated blood from the body, the heart immediately sends that blood over to the lungs. There, each inhalation we make serves to load that blood with oxygen (simultaneously, each exhalation sends carbon dioxide out of our body). The now-oxygenated blood is then immediately sent back to a different area of the heart that sends the blood out to the body through the aorta. A portion of the blood in the aorta is sent through two carotid arteries and two vertebral arteries which lead directly to the brain.

Upon reaching the brain, the carotid and vertebral arteries begin to separate, or 'branch', into smaller and smaller arteries. This can visually be represented by imagining how a large tree branch becomes smaller (and more branched) as it moves further away from the tree trunk. Eventually, the arteries delivering blood turn into capillaries which further branch out to the point that oxygen can be successfully delivered to every individual neuron within the brain.

As outlined previously, brain neurons have a relatively high metabolic rate and therefore require a constant supply of oxygen[3]. Like all cells, the brain cannot store oxygen within its tissue and consequently must receive a constant supply of oxygen from the bloodstream[20]. Even a few moments of inadequate blood supply to a neuron has the potential to disrupt normal cell function, but sustained disruption for just a few minutes leads to certain neuron death. Stroke is the end result of disrupted blood flow, and can be caused by either the leakage of blood from its vessel (i.e. 'hemorrhage'), or blockage of oxygenated blood that occurs from a clot.

Hemorrhage

In a healthy blood vessel, it is not possible for blood to escape from the vessel interior. Any evident leakage or flow of blood indicates that damage has occurred to that vessel. When blood is able to escape from a vessel, the process is known as *hemorrhage*. When hemorrhage occurs, cells further down the branching pathway of vessels from the area of hemorrhage are subjected to diminished or possibly ceased blood flow, a condition known as *ischemia*.

The hemorrhaging of blood from a vessel is proportionate to the size and type of blood vessel. Larger arteries carry a high rate of blood flow and the blood passes through the artery under a degree of pressure. Therefore, damage to an artery – particularly larger arteries – can result in a considerable amount of bleeding because of the pressure and rate of blood flow through arteries. Furthermore, it can take a significant amount of time to get arterial bleeding to stop – possibly even requiring surgical intervention. Capillary blood flow, on the other hand, exerts very little pressure. Capillaries have extremely thin walls and are densely packed in order to allow for the delivery and transfer of oxygen to every cell in their vicinity – so densely packed together, in fact, that the human body contains around 60,000 miles of blood vessels within its tissues[21], most of which are capillaries. In fact, over 1,000 miles of vessels exist just within the brain, most of which again are capillaries[22]. Hemorrhage to these capillaries has a slower release of blood than arteries but may result in considerable bleeding if enough capillaries are affected. After leaving the capillary, the blood enters into veins under minimal pressure compared to arteries. Still, injury such as an incision occurring to a vein may result in a sizeable amount of bleeding if the vein is of a larger size.

When vessels are damaged due to a wound on the surface of the skin, it is easily recognized as the blood pools or oozes from the wound. Internal hemorrhage, however, is much more difficult to recognize – especially in cases of spontaneous hemorrhage when no real suspicion for any injury has occurred. Stroke can result from spontaneous hemorrhage and is particularly problematic given that the brain is encased within the bony skull. This bony protection serves to safeguard the brain but can also make identification of the hemorrhage quite difficult. As such, recognizing brain hemorrhage can be dependent upon the patient first reporting symptoms capable of alerting a medical provider of the possibility of brain hemorrhage. Depending on factors such as the rate at which the bleeding occurs, development of hemorrhage-like symptoms in a patient may take some time which in turn results in delayed medical care – possibly to the point at which the hemorrhage has reached a life-threatening stage.

Clots

In addition to hemorrhage, a second way to prevent oxygenated blood from reaching the body's cells is through the development of a clot. A clot is a small mass of blood materials (e.g. platelets, proteins, etc.) that clump together within a vessel and consequently impede or halt blood flow through that vessel. Like hemorrhage, any cells further down a vessel from the clot will then be deprived of some or all oxygenated blood (i.e. will become *ischemic)* depending on how much blockage occurs.

In medical terms, the material comprising a clot within a vessel is known as a *thrombus,* and the process of clot formation is called *thrombosis.* Clots can form within the bloodstream due to multiple reasons[23], but typically occur in response to the body's normal process for

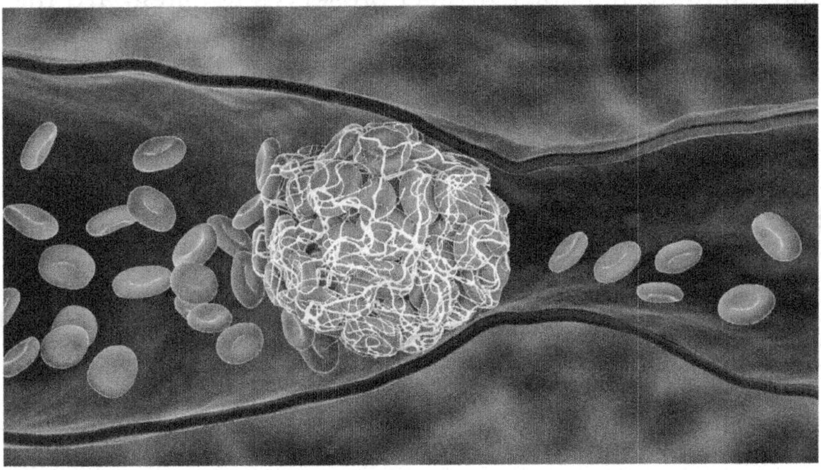

Figure 1.5. An embolism will continue to pass along an artery until it can no longer fit through, at which point it becomes lodged, occluding blood flow and preventing vital oxygen from reaching cells further down from the occlusion.

repairing damage to a blood vessel. If the clot remains in place during the repair and eventually dissolves after the repair is complete, no complications should be expected. However, clots do not always stay in place. In such cases, as the clot becomes dislodged and moves through the vessel it is known as an *embolism* or *thromboembolism.*

The material that makes up a clot is not problematic in itself given that it is created through a normal process that occurs within the body in response to vessel damage. Actually, clots are quite beneficial in that they exist to stop any leakage of blood when a vessel has been damaged. The bigger issue is that as the clot moves through an artery that delivers oxygenated blood, the artery's continuous branching creates arteries that are smaller and smaller in size. As these arteries becomes smaller, the area through which the blood passes – known as the 'lumen' – becomes smaller as well. Eventually, an embolism can reach an artery with a lumen small enough that the clot cannot pass through. In such a case, the clot becomes lodged within the artery creating what is known as an *occlusion* (see Figure 1.5). This occlusion plugs up the affected artery and prevents oxygenated blood from passing through, thereby creating an 'occluded artery'. Consequently, any cells (or neurons, in the specific case of stroke) awaiting oxygen further down from the occlusion become ischemic and will eventually die if the clot is not dislodged.

If the clot occurs within an artery of the brain, it is known as an ischemic stroke. If enough neurons die in response to the clot, there will be noticeable disruption to some body function depending upon which area of the brain is affected. As with hemorrhage, the amount of neurons susceptible to ischemia from an occluded artery is proportional to the size of the clot, as larger clots will occlude an artery earlier in the artery's 'branching', which in turn means that a higher number of smaller arteries awaiting blood from that blocked artery will fail to receive oxygenated blood. Consequently, a greater number of neurons will be at risk of cell death.

Summary

In this chapter we focused on outlining some of the fundamental concepts related to the brain's design, its organization, and its blood flow required to keep neurons alive. The neuron is the brain's specialized cell which gives us our ability to think, move, and recognize the world around us. Within the brain, neurons are linked together into regions that serve to coordinate and regulate specific body functions. The neurons within these regions must be continuously supplied with oxygen from the bloodstream, and any interruption to oxygen supply can result in neuronal death within minutes.

The material within this chapter provides an anatomical basis for the primary factors involved in stroke. Stroke itself results from an interruption to blood flow within the brain, and in understanding how the brain is designed and organized it allows us to build on these foundational concepts of the brain and begin to piece together the events involved in stroke. In the next chapter we will look at some of the intricacies of stroke including the types of stroke, how each type can occur, and some of the major statistics associated with each type of stroke.

Chapter 2 – Stroke

Stroke is unique in that it is a disease involving two major systems of the body – the cardiovascular system and the nervous system. The brain, a component of the nervous system, coordinates all the actions and processes that we as humans can perform. Despite the brain's amazing capabilities, its normal processes can quickly and permanently be jeopardized when complications arise through the cardiovascular system's interaction with the brain. Clots or hemorrhage within vessels of the cardiovascular system can cause death to neurons, which if occurring to a high enough degree can have debilitating consequences for the patient. In this chapter we'll build on our understanding of the brain and its associated blood flow to look specifically at the events involved in the development and occurrence of stroke – including how these events lead to the common signs and symptoms exhibited by many stroke patients.

Stroke

Stroke occurs when there is an abnormality in blood supply to the brain[24]. Adhering to this description, both a large vessel rupture within the brain or a microscopic occlusion of a single capillary qualify as stroke, though effects of the latter event may never even be realized. Because our understanding of stroke involves some degree of impairment to the patient, the World Health Organization defined stroke as *a clinical syndrome consisting of rapidly developing clinical signs of focal (or global in case of coma) disturbance of cerebral function lasting more than 24 hours or leading to death with no apparent cause other than a vascular origin*[25].

In simpler terms, stroke occurs when neurons within the brain are damaged due to a disruption of adequate oxygen delivery to those neurons[26]. As a disease, stroke has been classified as both a cardiovascular disease[27] as well as a neurological disease[28], but is commonly grouped under the larger umbrella of cardiovascular conditions such as coronary artery disease and deep vein thrombosis. Along with heart attack, stroke falls within the acute (i.e. 'rapid onset') grouping of cardiovascular diseases, and much like heart attack, stroke can have either fatal or recoverable outcomes depending upon its severity.

Stroke is the second leading cause of death worldwide after ischemic heart disease[29] and the fifth leading cause of death in the United States[30]. This is important to note, as stroke had previously been as high as 3rd on the list of leading causes of death in the United States. However, preventative efforts for stroke have been successful enough to move it down to 5th on the list[31]. Because of its effects, stroke is the most common source of long-term disability in adults[32], with 80% of its survivors expected to have some degree of permanent disability[33].

The word 'stroke' itself comes from the rapidness by which people are struck suddenly by the rapid onset of its effects[24]. These effects typically present few warning signs to the patient and as a result leave little opportunity for medical intervention to avert the stroke. Because of its debilitating effects, stroke is considered the most serious of the cerebrovascular diseases[31] – a group of conditions relating specifically to abnormal blood flow within the brain – though the actual degree of impairment after the stroke is dependent upon how long blood flow was disrupted as well as how much of the brain was affected.

Stroke statistics

Globally, nearly 17 million people suffer a stroke each year[34] and almost one in six individuals have a stroke in their lifetime[35]. Within the United States, over 600,000 individuals suffer an initial stroke annually while approximately 185,000 people experience a 'recurrent' stroke that occurs after having had an initial stroke[36].

These statistics equate to approximately one stroke incident every 40 seconds in the United States[36].

Though often associated with older age, nearly 1/3 of all strokes occur in patients who are less than 65 years old[37]. This contributes to over 7 million Americans aged 20 or older having had a stroke and nearly 3% of the population in the United States living with the effects of stroke[36]. These numbers result in costs associated with stroke now exceeding $70 billion annually[38] .

Specific to gender, The Centers for Disease Control have found that nearly 3% of both males and females report having a history of stroke[39] and as they advance in age, their likelihood of living with the effects of stroke also increase[36]. Females tend to have a lower stroke risk at a younger age than males, but females have a higher risk of stroke-related fatality than males[40]. Furthermore, stroke risk in females doubles in the decade following menopause, possibly due to metabolic changes such as increased blood pressure as well as alterations in body composition[41].

The gender differences in stroke risk are important to put into context. On average, females live longer than men. This in turn increases the length of time in which a stroke could occur, given that strokes are more likely to occur later in life and women tend to have a longer life expectancy. This increased life expectancy can in part explain why in the United States approximately 55,000 more women have a stroke than men[42]. Other potential factors for the higher occurrence of stroke in women include evidence that women tend to have higher blood pressure during pregnancy and report higher levels of stress than males[43]. Whereas increased age, elevated blood pressure, and stress are all risk factors for stroke, each of these measures may contribute to the higher overall rate of stroke occurrence in females.

Regarding ethnicity, stroke is lowest among Asians/Pacific Islanders at 1.8% and highest among American Indian/Alaska Natives at 5.4%, with other ethnicities falling within that range[36]. However, the risk for having an initial stroke is twice as high among African Americans as it is in Caucasians. Furthermore, in the United States, African Americans exhibit the highest rate of deaths due to stroke[43]. Still, the death rate from stroke has been on a decline among all ethnicities with the exception of Hispanics, who have seen a slight increase in stroke rate in the past decade[44].

Types of Stroke

Two predominant types of stroke occur: ischemic and hemorrhagic. Although the underlying causes of these two stroke types are very different, the outcome of each is similar in that the patient ultimately experiences blocked or suppressed blood flow to an area of their brain. Next, we will take a look at each type, highlighting the unique events involved in causing ischemic and hemorrhagic stroke.

Ischemic stroke

Ischemic stroke results when blood flow through an artery of the brain becomes blocked and subsequently causes death to some degree of brain cells, a situation known in medical terms as an *infarction*. Worldwide, about 68% of strokes are ischemic in nature[45] while in the United States that number is much higher at 87%[36]. A subtype of ischemic stroke is known as acute ischemic stroke and has been defined as *the development of sudden neurological deficits resulting from a focal injury due to vascular occlusion in the central nervous system*[46]. Most often, the blockage associated with acute ischemic stroke results from an embolism originating from outside the brain that eventually lodges itself within one of the brain's arteries[31].

Three types of acute ischemic stroke exist – large vessel stroke, small vessel stroke (i.e. 'Lacunar' stroke), and cardioembolic stroke[47]. A large vessel stroke occurs in response to a clot or blockage within the large arteries of the brain, while a small vessel stroke results from blockage within the brain's micro-vascular areas including the capillaries. Cardioembolic strokes result in blockage to a cerebral artery from a thrombus that originated specifically from within the heart tissue.

In addition to clots, ischemic strokes can be caused by cardiac-related issues such as atrial fibrillation or atherosclerosis[48]. Although atrial fibrillation is a term relating to abnormal heart rhythm, it can also result in the generation of clots within the heart's tissue[49]. These clots can escape the heart as an embolism and eventually lodge within an artery of the brain, resulting in ischemic stroke. Separately, atherosclerosis is the cause of nearly 20% of ischemic strokes[50]. Atherosclerosis and its associated plaque formation cause narrowing of arteries, and this narrowing is particularly problematic when occurring within the arteries of the brain. Disruption to these plaques can result in development of clots which subsequently detach and travel to the brain[51]. Identification of the source of ischemic stroke is important, as patients whose initial stroke was caused by atherosclerosis have a higher risk of suffering a later stroke – even when on medication to treat their initial stroke[52].

Transient ischemic attack

Any impaired flow of blood to the brain can loosely meet the definition of stroke. There is, however, a range of time which can determine whether that impaired blood flow is consequential to the patient. When blood flow to an area of the brain is decreased by up to half, the patient largely remains absent of any symptoms[31]. A further decrease, though, can initiate a range of symptoms that are dependent upon which area of the brain is affected. In cases where blood flow is quickly restored – such as when a clot that was partially occluding an artery ultimately dissolves – the patient has no lasting effects and will eventually return to normal. When that occurs, the patient is said to have experienced a *transient ischemic attack* (TIA), which essentially translates to a 'short period of diminished oxygen supply to the brain'. Officially defined as *a transient episode of neurologic dysfunction caused by focal brain ischemia without evidence of acute infarction on brain imaging,* the main difference between TIA and stroke is the degree of infarction – no tissue death occurs in the brain with TIA while a stroke by definition results in tissue death[53].

It might be said that a TIA is a sort of 'near stroke' that was resolved prior to the full events of stroke happening. Regardless, a TIA should be considered a warning sign and not ignored, especially in light of evidence revealing that experiencing a TIA increases one's risk of stroke[54]. However, the reported risk of stroke after TIA appears to have decreased in the past few decades[54] dropping from what was once as high as a 20% risk in the three months following a TIA to now just under 4%, or approximately one-sixth the risk previously reported[55]. This reduction in risk is thought to be the result of better post-stroke prevention strategies designed to help limit the risk of a second stroke. Despite the reduction, it is recommended that patients who experience a TIA make immediate lifestyle adjustments to ward off a future stroke – especially high-risk patients such as those of advanced age or who have high blood pressure[54].

Hemorrhagic stroke

Whereas ischemic stroke refers to the interruption of oxygenated blood to a portion of the brain, hemorrhagic stroke refers to bleeding in the brain due to a ruptured blood vessel. It is believed that hemorrhagic stroke is most commonly caused by chronic (i.e. 'long term') high blood pressure that weakens an area of vessels in the brain to the point where they eventually rupture[56]. Regarding severity, hemorrhagic stroke is considered much more life-threatening than ischemic stroke due to the potential for ongoing bleeding as well as increased blood pressure within the skull, and hemorrhagic stroke has a higher mortality rate after one month[57].

Worldwide, nearly one in three strokes are due to hemorrhage[45]; however, only around 10% of strokes occurring within the United States are hemorrhagic[36]. The most common sites in the brain for hemorrhagic stroke to occur are within the basal ganglia near the center of the brain (approximately 50% of hemorrhagic stroke events), followed by the cerebral lobes (10% to 20%), thalamus (15%), pons and the brain stem (10% to 20%), and the cerebellum (10%)[58].

Intracerebral Hemorrhage

Two types of hemorrhagic stroke have been identified. The first, intracerebral hemorrhage (ICH), is defined as *rapidly developing clinical signs of neurological dysfunction attributable to a focal collection of blood within the brain parenchyma or ventricular system that is not caused by trauma*[59]. In other words, ICH is the result of bleeding that occurs within the brain tissue (i.e. 'parenchyma') itself. Intracerebral hemorrhage can be quite damaging in nature, as research has revealed that less than 40% of patients who experience ICH are likely to achieve functional independence[60].

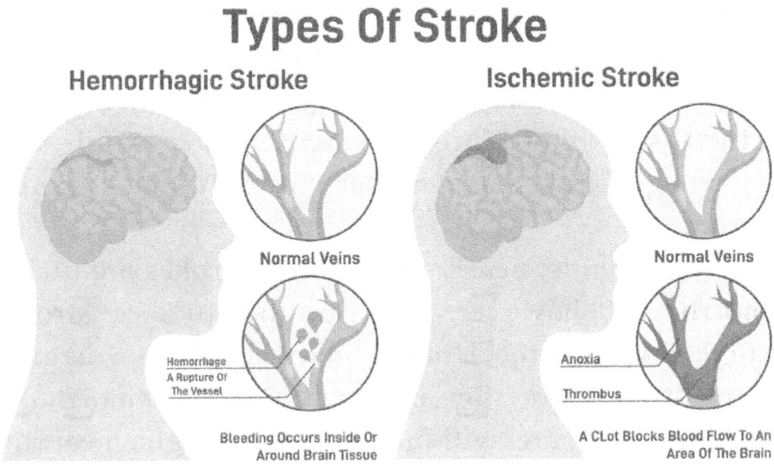

Figure 2.1. Hemorrhagic stroke - including intracerebral hemorrhage - results from the leakage of blood from an artery in the brain, while ischemic stroke occurs in response to an embolism (clot) that occludes blood flow within the brain.

Intracerebral hemorrhage can be categorized as traumatic or spontaneous. "Traumatic ICH" occurs in response to head trauma that then triggers bleeding within the brain. Spontaneous, or "non-traumatic ICH" is the form of ICH in which the bleeding occurs without warning in absence of any sort of head trauma and is considered the deadliest form of stroke[61]. Non-traumatic ICH causes nearly 15% of all strokes in the United States[62] with little improvement in these rates over the past few decades[60].

Non-traumatic ICH strokes can be further grouped as primary or secondary in nature. Primary ICH is the more common of the two forms (~60%)[63] and results when the hemorrhage is caused by chronic high blood pressure. This high blood pressure can create microscopic alterations within the vessel walls, eventually increasing the vessel's susceptibility to rupture[64]. Primary ICH can also result from amyloid angiopathy[65], a condition in which proteins accumulate within the walls of the arteries of the brain that subsequently weaken the artery itself[66,67]. Secondary ICH occurs in response to an existing blood vessel abnormality in the brain such as arteriovenous malformations or aneurysms[68], and occurs much less frequently than primary ICH[69, 70].

Intracerebral Hemorrhage Statistics

Over 63,000 cases of intracerebral hemorrhage occur in the United States annually, with global rates approximately 15% higher[71]. Reports indicate that ICH occurs at the highest rate (80%) in countries designated as low or middle-income[72], and the rate of ICH in these countries has not decreased over the years[72]. In contrast, rates of ICH have been shown to decrease in developed countries, thought to be due in part to better treatment and control of hypertension, a primary cause of ICH[73].

The increasing age of the global population suggests that the occurrence of ICH will increase 35% by the year 2050, along with a doubling of ICH cases in patients over 80 years of age[74]. Specific to age, it has been shown that the risk of ICH increases as an individual grows older such that six ICH strokes occur per 100,000 individuals aged 35-54 years. This rate goes up to 37.2 and 176.3 in those aged 55-74 and 75-94 years, respectively[75]. Using the same age-based comparison by gender, it was reported that males experience ICH more often than females, and the rates are again age-specific. Among males and females aged 35-54 years old, males had a rate of 5.9 ICH strokes per 100,000 individuals versus 5.1 in females. The rates climbed to 37.2 (males) and 26.4 (females) in the 55-74 year age group and 176.3 (males) versus 140.1 (females) in the 75-94 age group[75].

Subarachnoid Hemorrhage

The second type of hemorrhagic stroke is known as subarachnoid hemorrhage (SAH) which comprises approximately 3% of strokes that occur in the United States[36]. Subarachnoid hemorrhage stroke results from *rapidly developing signs of neurological dysfunction and/or headache because of bleeding into the subarachnoid space (the space between the arachnoid membrane and the pia mater of the brain or spinal cord), which is not caused by trauma*[59].

Because the bleeding occurs in the space formed between the brain and bony skull, SAH causes a dual crisis for patients. First, the hemorrhage prevents an area of neurons in the brain from receiving vital oxygen. Secondly, continued bleeding into the brain can cause a pooling of blood that if not addressed immediately, can become particularly problematic.

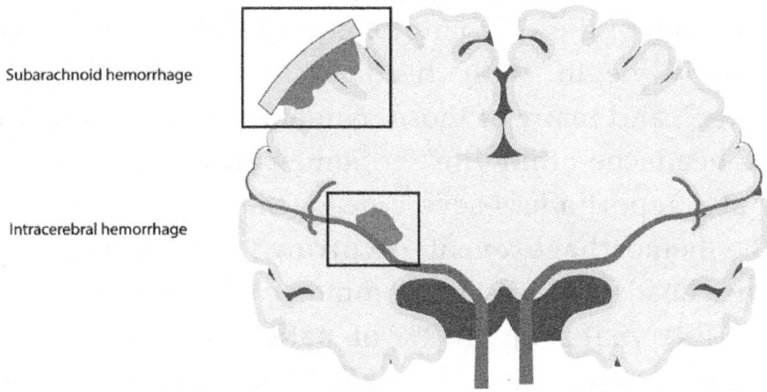

Figure 2.2. Whereas intracerebral hemorrhage occurs within the brain tissue, subarachnoid hemorrhage results when blood pools between the brain tissue and the bony skull.

With the brain being surrounded by the bony skull, blood that escapes from the brain cannot settle into the surrounding tissue. Consequently, blood pooling within the skull begins to build up and compress the brain tissue itself. This compression can have detrimental effects for the patient due to diminished blood flow to the brain as well as causing deformation of the brain itself, and the compression can impact cellular events that ultimately impede neuron metabolism and signaling activity[56], all of which can result in a life-threatening situation for the patient.

Subarachnoid hemorrhage can be brought about by a range of conditions including physical activity or psychological stress[76]. In 80% of cases, SAH is caused by the rupture of an existing aneurysm, though SAH can also be caused by inflammation or blood vessel malformations within the brain[77]. Symptoms associated with SAH commonly begin with headache in nearly 60% of patients[78], and many of those patients report having "the worst headache of my life"[79]. Some patients (up to 40%) may also report a less-severe headache in the days prior to the hemorrhage event occurring[80]. Unfortunately, because headache is itself a common cause for emergency room (ER) visits (up to 2% of patients)[81] and is more frequently observed in the ER than those headaches resulting specifically from SAH (less than 1% of ER-associated headaches), the early symptoms of SAH including headache may be misdiagnosed in the ER as a migraine. Such cases may regrettably result in no beneficial treatment being provided for the SAH patient[82,83].

Among SAH patients who received no treatment, their mortality rate reached 50-65% in the year following their stroke. With effective medical care, this rate can be reduced to as low as 18%[60, 84, 85]. Such evidence clearly indicates the importance of early recognition of SAH as well as proper treatment. Still, the long-term effects of

SAH are problematic, as patients tend to have significant disability after 1 year[86].

Subarachnoid Hemorrhage Statistics

The occurrence rate of SAH is approximately 5 events per 100,000 individuals[87], and like ischemic stroke, SAH rates are higher in lower-income countries[88]. It is suspected that the true rates for SAH are even higher given that up to 15% of patients who experience SAH do not make it to the hospital[88]. Though disheartening, it is helpful to know that mortality rates for SAH have been falling approximately 1% per year since the mid-1970s[89] thanks to improved treatment[88] along with an overall decrease in smoking rates[90].

As it relates to age and occurrence, SAH strokes have a tendency to occur in patients of a younger age than those who suffer ischemic stroke[91]. Specific to gender, females suffer SAH at a higher rate (65%) than males[87]. Based on ethnicity, Mexican-Americans have been found to be most susceptible to suffering SAH[92].

Effects of stroke on the neuron

Regardless of which type of stroke a patient experiences, the end effect of stroke is a deprivation of oxygen to an area of the brain which ultimately results in the death of neurons. When neuronal death within the brain happens, several structural and metabolic changes occur. Neurons directly in the area deprived of oxygen experience a phenomenon known as *liquefactive necrosis* whereby the neurons are eventually eliminated by the body over a period of months[93, 94].

Those neurons not directly impacted by the process of necrosis can exhibit swelling or may undergo structural alterations, conditions which indicate damage to the neuron. However, if the damage is not extensive, there is a chance that the neuron can recover to some degree[43]. In the hours and days following stroke, the progression of this neuronal damage is critical to control. Dead neurons in the brain cannot regenerate and therefore any body functions regulated by those neurons are permanently lost[95]. In order to limit the progression of damage, one of the main goals in stroke management has long been to save as many of the 'recoverable' neurons as possible[96].

Immediately after the stroke event, there is evidence of inflammatory cell presence in both the ischemic area and the surrounding area[97]. The fact that inflammatory cells can be found in the affected area indicates that the patient's autoimmune system recognizes that some degree of damage has occurred. This activation of the immune system can bring additional complications to the area such as a potential for swelling – which can be problematic given the limited space within the skull[98] – along with a variety of other chemical and physical cellular events.

Common signs and symptoms of stroke

As we have seen, the degree of impairment that a patient experiences as a result of stroke is dependent upon the location of the stroke within the brain as well as the overall extent of blood flow blockage or hemorrhage that occurs. Recognizing that a stroke has occurred is largely dependent upon the recognition of signs and symptoms indicative of stroke which alerts the patient or others (e.g. friends, family, bystanders, etc.) that a stroke is occurring. Recognizing the signs and symptoms of stroke is vital, since – as we will discuss in detail later – any delay in care can have significant consequences for the patient.

Because stroke can occur effectively anywhere within the brain, there could exist such a vast number of signs and symptoms that it would easily be possible to say that literally 'anything' abnormal about the patient could be indicative of stroke. Still, there are certain signs and symptoms that are more common in a stroke patient and should key in those who know or are around the patient as to the possibility of stroke. The most commonly reported signs and symptoms of stroke can include 'drooping' of the face, asymmetrical (non-equal) facial expressions, sudden weakness or numbness in a limb or on one side of the body, headache, confusion, vision issues or visual field disturbances, trouble speaking or swallowing, sudden memory issues, or difficulty understanding speech[99-101].

It has also been reported that certain symptoms are more commonly associated with a certain stroke type. For example, one study found that dilated pupils, agitation of the patient, sudden headache, and seizure were more common to hemorrhagic stroke patients, while a slowly progressing headache was more indicative of ischemic stroke[102]. It should be noted, though, that recognizing the likelihood of symptoms being associated with a particular type of stroke is largely the responsibility of medical professionals for situations where medical imaging may not be readily available. For the overall health of the patient, the priority should be on identifying *any* symptoms which could be indicative of stroke and getting that patient to advanced medical care.

Stroke in the age of COVID-19

The global pandemic of 2020 taught us new ways to live, to interact, and to try and stay healthy. Despite using masks and social distancing precautions, many of us continue to deal with wave after wave of COVID-19 exposures and infections. One of the early characteristics we learned about COVID-19 was that it tended to have the most impact on those individuals with other existing medical issues such as obesity, heart conditions, or other significant medical problems. Given the debilitating effects that stroke can have, it is important to recognize a stroke patient's risk potential specific to COVID-19.

Research indicates that there is not yet a clear relationship between stroke and COVID-19 in that COVID-19 does not appear to cause stroke and stroke does not show evidence of making a patient more susceptible to COVID-19[103]. Researchers have, however, shown that an individual's stroke risk during the pandemic was indeed higher if they had cardiovascular risk factors such as hypertension[103]. Still, an important stroke-related concern was revealed when researching viruses. Specifically, researchers found that there is a 7.6 times higher odds of developing stroke after COVID-19 compared with influenza[103]. Unfortunately, a conclusive reason explaining this higher risk was not found.

Conclusion

Understanding the basics of stroke can help patients and caregivers appreciate the vast range of effects that stroke can bring. Stroke is either ischemic or hemorrhagic in nature, and has several subtypes within those two classifications. The severity of a patient's stroke is dependent upon a variety of factors but largely comes down to the location and degree of occlusion within the brain. Therefore, because stroke can occur effectively anywhere in the brain, two patients diagnosed with stroke may have vastly different signs and symptoms. In the next chapter we'll discuss some of the stroke risk factors that when present can predispose an individual to having a stroke. Understanding risk factors can help patients become more aware of their own risks and allow those patients to engage in practices which can help reduce their risk of suffering a stroke.

Chapter 3 – Risk Factors for Stroke

When medical professionals evaluate risk, they look at certain characteristics of a person which can increase or decrease that person's likelihood of experiencing a certain medical condition. Those characteristics are considered 'factors', and when those factors increase a patient's chance of experiencing a disease they are known as *risk factors*. The more risk factors a person has, the more likely that same person is to experience a certain medical condition whether it be a skin condition, bone fracture, or stroke.

Risk is considered as an assessment of the possibility of harm. In medicine, the 'possibility' is represented as the likelihood of experiencing the particular illness or injury. For most injuries or illness, there is always some risk of occurrence, and thankfully there are almost always opportunities to reduce the risk of that injury or illness from occurring. Walking out of your house, for example, invites the possibility of rolling your ankle, or catching pneumonia, or being hit in the head by a falling branch. While these situations may seem minimal or even absurd in some cases, they do exist. Oftentimes, decisions we make as individuals can serve to amplify or even decrease our risk of such situations happening. For example, holding on to a handrail as we walk down our front steps can reduce the risk of rolling our ankle. Wearing a mask or avoiding public places reduces our risk of contracting pneumonia. Keeping trees trimmed or not going outside during a storm reduces our risk of being hit by a branch. Despite seeming obvious at times, risk is not always so evident nor is it always easy to avoid.

Stroke, like contracting pneumonia or getting hit by a branch, has associated risks which increase or decrease its likelihood of occurrence. Because of stroke's severe and debilitating effects, it is important for individuals to try and minimize as many risk factors as possible. As we will discuss, reducing stroke risk is not always easy since some risk factors like gender or age cannot be altered. Other risk factors such as having high cholesterol may go undetected. In this chapter we will outline many of the most common risk factors for stroke and also discuss how risk factors can influence an individual's likelihood of having a second stroke. First, however, we will explore risk factors in general to help you understand their different types as well as how they are determined.

Risk Factors

Risk factors can be grouped several different ways. One option is to separate risk factors into 'modifiable' and 'non-modifiable' where the grouping is based upon an individual's influence over that risk factor. Modifiable risk factors are those which the affected individual can alter. For example, high consumption of saturated fat is a known risk factor for heart disease. Because an individual can control the amount of saturated fat they consume, high saturated fat intake is considered a modifiable risk factor for cardiovascular disease. Age is also a risk factor for cardiovascular disease since older age increases one's risk for cardiovascular events such as a heart attack. Unfortunately, it is not possible to voluntarily decrease one's age; therefore, age is considered a 'non-modifiable' risk factor. In most cases, non-modifiable risk factors simply cannot be avoided and the individual has to accept the inherent risk.

Another way risk factors can be grouped is by separating them into 'extrinsic' and 'intrinsic' risk. With this method, the grouping of risk is determined by the individual's ability to control the risk. Extrinsic risk factors are similar to modifiable risk factors in that they can be altered by the individual. With heart attack risk, extrinsic factors could include smoking, obesity, or physical inactivity which, if changed in a favorable way would reduce that individual's risk for heart attack. Conversely, intrinsic risk factors are those which are inherent to the individual and cannot be changed. Examples of intrinsic risk factors include age, gender, or having a family history of coronary artery disease, among others.

The final way risk factors can be grouped is through the 'behavioral' classification. Typically, behavioral risk factors are actions which are considered unhealthy in nature and can be changed. Examples of behavioral risk factors can include smoking, inactivity, or excess alcohol consumption. As you might have noticed, behavioral risk factors are similar in nature to both extrinsic and modifiable risk factors in that they are largely under some level of control by the patient. Nonbehavioral risk factors could include age, gender, or geographical location, and are related somewhat to intrinsic and non-modifiable risk factors.

Simply speaking, the goal for any individual is to reduce as many modifiable, extrinsic, or behavioral risk factors as possible. This in turn leaves only the non-modifiable or intrinsic risk factors as contributing to one's risk for experiencing a specific medical condition. Next, let's address how risk factors are determined through the study of populations. Understanding how risk factors are developed can help you understand why stroke happens and can also help you better recognize how to reduce the risk of an additional (i.e. 'recurrent') stroke.

Determining Risk

Unfortunately, in order to improve our understanding of stroke, strokes have to occur. Medicine can then study those stroke events and try to learn something from each while also adding information about that stroke to a larger database. Good data must come from a wide range of patients of various age, ethnicities, weight, activity level, dietary habits, family medical histories, and more, and these same categories must consist of people who have and have not experienced stroke. As more strokes happen over time – which may take decades – enough data points are generated that we can then recognize 'trends' in the data. These trends start to identify risk and inform us about how a particular medical condition or illness affects a specific population.

It should be emphasized that risk factors are based on the *likelihood* of a certain characteristic (e.g. smoking) contributing to a medical event's occurrence – they do not guarantee that the event will occur. In other words, even though an individual may have several risk factors, he or she may never experience the event in question. For example, a 72-year-old individual who is inactive, smokes a pack of cigarettes per day, and eats fast-food six nights a week has several risk factors for cardiovascular disease. Still, he may go his whole life without a cardiac-related medical event. On the opposite side, a 48-year-old non-smoker who runs 30 miles per week and eats a balanced diet could experience a heart attack despite having very few risk factors. So many variables are at play in every individual that it can be difficult to narrow down risk to just one or two factors. For example, having a family history of heart disease can trump the fact that the 48-year-old individual was a non-smoker and a runner, thereby making him or her at a higher risk for cardiovascular disease than the 72-year-old individual. Again, risk factors determine likelihood based on a set of characteristics about the individual, but do not guarantee an event will occur.

Before diving into the risk factors of stroke, we have to discuss one final concept – *comorbidity*. Comorbidity, sometimes listed as a 'comorbid condition', is the existence of a second (or third, or fourth) medical condition which could affect, complicate, or worsen the severity of the first. For example, long-term high cholesterol increases one's risk for coronary artery disease. If a person with high cholesterol has high blood pressure at the same time – the high blood pressure would be considered a comorbidity and therefore further increase his or her risk for coronary artery disease than just high cholesterol alone as his or her heart is working harder (as evidenced by the elevated blood pressure) while also at risk for being provided less oxygen necessary to pump correctly (due to the risk of plaque buildup within the coronary artery as is common with high cholesterol). Comorbidities can complicate the patient's overall medical status, and in some cases may even interfere with the patient's medical care in cases where treatment for one condition could negatively impact the second condition.

Comorbidities play a major role in stroke and stroke risk. For example, a person who smokes is at increased risk for stroke, but if they have a comorbid condition of high blood pressure their risk for stroke increases immensely. As we will see next, stroke has many associated risk factors. Some of these factors such as diabetes or high cholesterol can go unseen, which emphasizes the importance of regular physical examinations. Though we haven't yet been able to decipher the intricacies of why certain people of varying risk develop – or do not develop – stroke, rest assured that medical researchers are working to find out.

Risk factors for stroke

Stroke is considered a cardiovascular disease, and therefore most – but not all – cardiovascular risk factors have some level of influence on stroke risk. Globally speaking, 91% of one's risk for stroke can be linked to modifiable risk factors including high blood pressure, obesity, elevated blood sugar (i.e. hyperglycemia), elevated blood fats (hyperlipidemia), and kidney issues. Approximately 74% of an individual's stroke risk is attributed to behavioral risk factors such as smoking, living a sedentary lifestyle, or consumption of an unhealthy diet[104]. Similarly, a large study from the

United States looking at over 110,000 individuals found that unhealthy behaviors such as smoking, excess alcohol use, physical inactivity, and a poor diet accounted for half of the study participants' accumulated stroke risk. The same study revealed that participants who utilized healthy lifestyle choices such as not smoking, maintaining a healthy weight, and engaging in daily physical activity reduced their stroke risk by 80%[105].

These research findings specific to modifiable and behavioral risk factors are of extreme importance given that they highlight that an individual's stroke risk can be significantly reduced by making healthy choices. While non-modifiable risk factors such as family history or gender are also at play, these and other non-modifiable risk factors have less influence on one's stroke risk than modifiable risk factors. The basis behind as to how some of these conditions relate to stroke risk is discussed next.

Non-modifiable risk factors

Non-modifiable risk factors, or more specifically 'risk markers', are characteristics inherent to an individual which cannot be changed but may play a role in that person's risk for a particular disease. Several risk markers can factor into an individual's stroke risk. Although these risk markers are genetic and therefore considered non-modifiable, it is important to understand their involvement in order to help potentially recognize one's risk of suffering from stroke.

Age

Stroke has been called "a disease of aging"[106]. The average age at which ischemic stroke occurs is 69.2 years while hemorrhagic stroke seems to occur most frequently around 65 years of age[107]. Unfortunately, the older an individual gets, the more their stroke risk increases, with that risk eventually doubling each decade after the age of 55[108].

Gender

Stroke risk between males and females is dependent upon the patient's age. Among younger patients, females are at a slightly higher risk of stroke. It is suspected that this increased risk in women is due to pregnancy-related risk as well as potential hormone-related factors such as can occur in response to contraceptive use[108]. At older ages the risk of stroke increases for men[108], though after age 85 the risk appears to become equal[109] or slightly higher for women[110].

This shift in risk for women as they get older might seem odd, but remember from the prior chapter that women tend to live longer than men. Therefore, since advanced age is associated with increased stroke risk, women living longer than men tends to result in more women ultimately suffering stroke compared to men.

Ethnicity

Stroke risk has been shown to differ based on ethnicity, and minority groups consistently show higher stroke rates than Caucasian Americans[111]. The highest risk for ischemic stroke is within the American Indian group, who have stroke rates that exceed all other ethnicities[111]. African-Americans are at twice the risk of having a first stroke compared to Caucasians, and African-Americans under the age of 65 have up to five times the risk of stroke[112]. Furthermore, Hispanics have a higher risk than white non-Hispanic individuals[113] while Asian-Americans have been shown to be more at-risk for severe ischemic stroke than Caucasians[114].

Genetics

There are known genetic factors that play a role in stroke risk. Family history is often cited as a risk for stroke, but consideration of one's genetics more specifically outlines their risk. Family history risk is itself tied more in with the individual's home environment such as dietary habits, exposure to cigarette smoke, or daily physical activity levels[106], each of which can be its own risk factor. Genetic risk, on the other hand, is specific to the percent of risk that is inherited from one's parents[115] and is largely tied to the patient's risk for blood coagulation issues as well as their risk for atrial fibrillation.

Modifiable risk factors

Physical Inactivity

Physical inactivity is itself associated with multiple risk factors for stroke including elevated cholesterol, obesity, and diabetes. Stroke risk is also tied in with physical inactivity, though it is not clear in the research whether increased physical activity influences stroke directly or whether physical activity influences other stroke-related risk factors such as blood pressure or excess body weight[106].

High blood pressure

As a modifiable risk factor, one's blood pressure level has a strong association to stroke risk in that higher blood pressure values increase risk while normal blood pressure reduces stroke risk. Blood pressure measurements are comprised of two numbers and is commonly stated as "180 over 90", of which the first number (i.e. 'diastolic') represents how forcefully the heart contracts and the second number ('systolic') indicates how much the heart relaxes between contractions. Higher diastolic numbers – typically those readings above 130 – indicate that the heart is contracting with increased force in order to pump blood. That forceful pumping then strains the blood vessels, including the relatively sensitive blood vessels of the brain. In the case of hemorrhagic stroke, long-term high blood pressure can damage those sensitive vessels and eventually trigger the characteristic bleeding within the brain.

Long-term elevated blood pressure, known medically as 'hypertension' is commonly cited as the most common *modifiable* risk factor for both ischemic and hemorrhagic strokes. Most medical recommendations will state that 'normal' blood pressure is indicated by a reading of 120/80 mM Hg. Stroke risk appears to be reduced significantly by achieving a blood pressure reading at or below 130/80 mM Hg – slightly higher than normal but much lower than problematic values such as 180/100 mM Hg or higher[116].

With stroke risk, the systolic value appears to be more relevant than the diastolic value[117]. Specifically, a systolic number below 130 has been recommended as a viable goal for reducing one's risk of stroke. While studies have shown that reducing high blood pressure has an important influence on reducing an individual's risk for stroke[118], attempting to reduce blood pressure well below a range of 'normal' does not result in an additional decrease in stroke risk[119].

Diabetes

Diabetes is a medical condition in which the body is unable to properly process sugar. Individuals with diabetes have been reported to have a 50% higher chance of stroke than individuals without diabetes. The rationale for this higher risk is not well understood but it is suspected to be linked at least in part to atherosclerosis brought about by insulin resistance[120].

Dietary Intake

Traditionally, a well-balanced diet designed around preventing excess caloric intake is recommended for a healthy lifestyle. With stroke, however, Mediterranean-style diets have specifically been recommended and are generally successful in reducing stroke risk[121], and that risk appears to apply to both ischemic and hemorrhagic stroke[122]. Furthermore, Mediterranean diets can reduce stroke risk by over 40% in high-risk patients shown to be at increased risk for stroke[123]. Mediterranean diets emphasize plant-based foods including fruits and vegetables, whole grains, legumes and nuts, along with an emphasis of olive oil as a fat in place of butter or vegetable oil. In addition, Mediterranean diets recommend herbs and spices rather than table salt for seasoning, thereby also helping to reduce the stroke patient's sodium intake. Based on the success Mediterranean-style diets have shown for reducing stroke risk, policy-making organizations commonly recommend stroke patients adopt Mediterranean-style diets[124].

Cholesterol level

Chronically high circulating blood lipids such as triglycerides or cholesterol are associated with an increased stroke risk. In terms of cholesterol, using medication to decrease one's low-density lipoprotein (LDL, often reported as 'bad cholesterol') levels had a beneficial effect on decreasing one's risk of stroke[125] as well as reducing the risk of a recurrent stroke[126].

Obesity

Much like physical activity and stroke risk, the research related to obesity is not consistent on whether obesity alone influences stroke risk or whether other medical conditions occurring in conjunction with obesity – such as high blood pressure or elevated cholesterol – are to blame. One study reported that overweight individuals are at higher risk for stroke, and the risk increases for each 5 kilograms of body weight an individual maintains[127]. Still, much of the risk in these obese individuals could be accounted for by the comorbidities of hypertension, elevated cholesterol, and elevated glucose levels[128].

Abdominal obesity has been called out as a risk factor for ischemic stroke[129]. Still, other research has indicated no association between obesity and stroke risk despite study participants having significant risk for other cardiovascular diseases[130]. However, research has indicated that weight loss itself can be associated with decreased cardiovascular risk, including the risk specific to stroke[131].

Smoking

Smoking has a strong association with stroke risk, though the reason for the increased risk is not well known. A large study found that smokers were 60% more likely to suffer a stroke than non-smokers, and even former smokers who have since quit maintained a higher stroke risk than non-smokers[132]. Researchers estimated that an individual's stroke risk increases by 12% for each increment of 5 cigarettes per day; therefore, an individual who smokes one pack (20 cigarettes) per day increases his or her stroke risk by almost 50%, while someone smoking two packs per day effectively doubles their initial stroke risk. The same study also reported that compared to non-smokers, female smokers had a higher risk for stroke than male smokers.

Unfortunately, even ongoing secondhand smoke exposure is problematic and increases one's stroke risk by 30-45%[132, 133]. In addition, elderly patients with a history of smoking are at increased risk of stroke recurrence compared to the risk found in non-smoking elderly patients[134].

Reducing the risk of stroke recurrence

Once the initial stroke has been stabilized, attention turns toward how to prevent additional strokes from occurring. For those patients who do suffer a second stroke, evidence suggests that it will most likely be the same type of stroke as the first[135]. It has been estimated that approximately 11% of stroke patients will have a second stroke within a year and 26% of patients will have a recurrent stroke within 5 years[135]. Prevention of recurrent stroke is important, especially since a patient's functional status after a recurrent stroke is frequently worse than after the original stroke[136].

In general, prevention of stroke recurrence focuses on eliminating or reducing existing risk factors in conjunction with lifestyle modifications[137]. Techniques to reduce risk factors may require actions on the part of the patient (e.g. improved diet, increased physical activity level, etc.) and potentially the use of certain medications like statins and anti-coagulants to reduce cardiac-related risk factors[138,139]. The American Heart Association acknowledges that lifestyle changes such as increasing one's physical activity level or cessation of smoking can be difficult, but the likelihood of success is often increased when the individual receives interactive counseling on how to incorporate these lifestyle changes[124]. Therefore, it is important for patients and caregivers to seek and/or receive appropriate counseling in order to increase their likelihood of success.

Depression is known to occur after stroke, and is considered the most common psychological problem after the initial stroke[140]. Stroke survivors who suffer from depression are at increased risk of worse functional recovery, diminished quality of life, and have a higher mortality rate than non-depressed patients[141]. Furthermore, depression after an initial stroke has been shown to increase a patient's risk of recurrent stroke as well[142]. Therefore, reducing the risk of a second stroke should focus not only on reducing known risk factors but also attempt to address existing depression.

Conclusion

As a disease, stroke has a variety of associated risk factors that can increase an individual's susceptibility to suffering a stroke. Many of these risk factors can be reduced through changes an individual makes to their lifestyle such as improved diet, cessation of smoking, or increasing their physical activity levels. Other non-modifiable risk factors such as age, gender, or family history cannot be changed. To reduce stroke risk, it is recommended that individuals eliminate as many modifiable risk factors as possible. Those patients who do suffer a stroke can reduce their risk of a recurrent stroke by eliminating or reducing many of the same risk factors. In the next chapter we will shift from the underlying basis and risks of stroke and begin focusing on stroke occurrence by outlining stroke 'mimics', which are a variety of medical conditions that can initially appear as stroke but are in fact separate medical conditions.

Chapter 4 – Stroke Mimics

It might seem like an odd title for a chapter, but stroke 'mimics' are a very important aspect of the stroke diagnosis process. Mimics are those medical conditions which present similarly to stroke but are in fact a separate disease. You can find mimics across all medical conditions, such as COVID-19 appearing like the flu and allergies possibly mimicking the common cold. Mimics are important for the medical team to be aware of when going through any diagnostic process, as being attentive to similar diseases can help prevent the team from having 'tunnel vision' and ultimately misdiagnosing the actual medical condition. Misdiagnoses can lead to incorrect treatments, which ultimately lead to a continuation of the existing medical problem since it is not being treated.

Though stroke mimics are not of direct concern for you as a patient or caregiver, it can be helpful to recognize some of the stroke mimics as they may be discussed while going through the initial phases of diagnosing stroke. In fact, the possibility of stroke mimics are the reason patients often receive an array of tests during the early stages of evaluation, as these tests both help to 'rule in' stroke as well as 'rule out' other medical conditions. Stroke has quite a few mimics which can include seizures, brain tumors, metabolic disorders, infectious conditions, psychological disorders, migraines, and nerve disorders among a variety of other medical conditions[143]. Therefore, this chapter is designed to provide you some information related to the most common stroke mimics as you may hear some of these conditions mentioned throughout the diagnostic process.

Seizures

Seizures occur when there is disrupted electrical activity in either the entire brain (i.e. "generalized" seizure) or a portion of the brain (i.e. "focal" seizure). Signs and symptoms of seizure include muscle weakness and/or paralysis, jerking-type movements, and having difficulty with walking. Additional symptoms of seizure can include a loss of consciousness and subsequent confusion upon waking, muscle spasms, drooling, clenching of the teeth, or rapid and uncontrolled eye movements[144].

Migraine

Migraine is a common headache disorder affecting around 11% of adults globally[145]. At present, the true cause of migraine remains undetermined, but it is suspected to be of neurological or vascular origin[146,147]. Migraine symptoms commonly include intense pain on one side of the head along with possible nausea and vomiting as well as a sensitivity to light and sound[148].

Brain tumors

Brain tumors are a relatively common form of cancer that occurs within the brain[149]. Tumors of the brain can come in many forms including gliomas (the most common type), astrocytomas, oligodendrogliomas, and schwannomas, among others[150]. Tumors can form in a variety of locations within the brain and cause symptoms that may include headache, nausea and vomiting, personality changes, irritability, or drowsiness, among many other symptoms[151].

Vestibular Dysfunction

The vestibular system helps us maintain balance by coordinating input from nerve sensors located throughout the body which provide the brain with information specific to the body's position. Patients experiencing a disruption of the vestibular system can lose orientation and struggle to perform common tasks such as walking or even standing upright. Symptoms of vestibular dysfunction include nausea, vomiting, vertigo, intolerance to head motion, uncontrolled and rapid eye movement, and postural instability[152].

Bell's Palsy

Stroke may occur in an area of the brain which affects functions of the head such as swallowing, speech, or facial movements. Bell's palsy is a condition in which the facial nerve itself is damaged. The facial nerve is responsible for our ability to make facial expressions but also has a role in taste and even our ability to produce tears. Patients suffering from Bell's palsy may experience facial 'drooping' or even one-sided facial paralysis including an inability to smile. In fact, Bell's palsy is the second-most common cause of one-sided facial paralysis behind only stroke[153]. Bell's palsy itself is not generally life-threatening in nature and most patients make a full recovery[154]. However, the similar presentation between Bell's palsy and stroke necessitates quick evaluation by a medical professional in order to determine which condition is responsible for the patient's signs and symptoms.

Subdural Hematoma

Pooling of blood between the brain and skull can occur as a result of head trauma or can occur without a known cause[155]. The resulting hematoma is particularly problematic because like those intracerebral hematomas associated with stroke, the increased pooling of blood that occurs in conjunction with subdural hematoma can compress or push against the brain to the point that normal brain activity is compromised. If occurring to a great enough degree, this compression can be life-threatening. Symptoms of subdural hematoma include headache, nausea and vomiting, alterations in mental status, seizure, gait abnormality, and possibly coma[156].

Dementia

Dementia is a collective term for a variety of conditions that cause an impaired ability to think, concentrate, remember, or make decisions, and can interfere with performing normal everyday activities. Because dementia encompasses a variety of medical conditions, there is not a singular origin for the patient's symptoms but rather a variety of causes including blood clots, immune response, plaque formation within nerves, or even stroke itself[157,158]. Symptoms of dementia can include increased difficulty with memory, attention, or communication, along with potential difficulty with reasoning, judgment, and problem solving. Patients in the early stages of dementia may also easily forget the name of close loved ones, get lost in familiar surroundings, fail to complete tasks, or speak somewhat incoherently[159].

Metabolic conditions

Like dementia, metabolic conditions that can appear similar to stroke are many and can include anything from electrolyte imbalance to hypoglycemia[160]. Causes for metabolic stroke mimics can include improper diet, overexertion, dehydration, or the existence of an underlying disease such as if the person is experiencing diabetic coma. Blood work performed upon the patient's arrival to the hospital can help eliminate or identify the likelihood of metabolic dysfunction. Symptoms of metabolic dysfunction can be wide-ranging but may include nausea, dizziness, fatigue, sluggishness, irritability, nervousness, or anxiety, among others.

Transient global amnesia

Typically occurring in older age, transient global amnesia (TGA) is the unexpected and sudden loss of recent memory. Typically, TGA is relatively short-lived and the patient's memory returns within the following 24 hours[161]. Patients with TGA will likely exhibit memory loss but otherwise have intact cognitive functions. Symptoms of TGA include the loss of recent memory and possibly some degree of confusion, which may result in the patient asking repetitive questions. The patient may also be anxious and possibly agitated. Upon the return of his or her memory, the patient may report some degree of memory loss around the time when the TGA was occurring[162].

Conclusion

The stroke mimics discussed in this chapter represent only the most common medical conditions which present similarly to stroke. In actuality, there are many more stroke mimics, most of which are less common than those listed in this chapter such as Wernicke's encephalopathy, Lyme neuroborreliosis, myasthenia gravis, Wegener's granulomatosis, or giant cell arteritis[163]. Although stroke may be suspected early upon arrival to the hospital and will often be the likely diagnosis, the stroke care team will still take their time and work together to evaluate for the likelihood of these mimics to ensure proper treatment is provided for the right condition. As a patient or caregiver, the initial minutes and hours of stroke care can be a dizzying array of tests, pokes and prods, along with shuffling the patient from one room to the next, all in an attempt to both identify stroke and rule out the likelihood of any of the stroke mimics. In the next chapter we will move to the diagnostic phase of stroke care and detail some of the processes commonly used to determine that a stroke has occurred. There can be quite a lot of tests and procedures performed during the diagnostic process, and it can be helpful to you to understand both what is occurring and the underlying basis for the many procedures.

Chapter 5 – Diagnosing Stroke

Diagnosis is the process of confirming an existing medical condition in a patient. Typically, diagnosis involves three steps including information about the patient and what they are experiencing, a physical examination, and finally diagnostic testing. Sometimes diagnosing a medical condition can be quite simple and requires only a visual examination, such as when diagnosing a skin rash. Other times, a tedious and involved array of evaluation and testing procedures are needed to establish the presence of a complex disease. Such is often the case for medical conditions such as stroke which cannot be easily observed and may leave a patient unable to describe what they are feeling.

Stroke is a relatively common condition within hospital emergency departments. As such, hospital medical teams are well-trained at caring for patients who arrive with the signs and symptoms of stroke. Although stroke is a common condition within emergency rooms, it can at times be difficult to recognize. Even when an initial suspicion of stroke exists, the similarity of stroke to its mimics such as head injury or even migraine can require an array of medical tests and procedures to confirm a diagnosis of stroke. Although going through medical test after medical test can be frustrating and perhaps even painful at times, it serves an important purpose – to ensure that the correct diagnosis is found.

In this chapter, we'll outline some of the most common procedures used in the process of diagnosing stroke in order to help you understand why the tests are used and what information the tests can provide. It should be noted that topics covered in this chapter are by no means a complete list of diagnostic procedures. Each facility's medical team will have their own evaluation and diagnostic protocol for suspected stroke, and the medical tests utilized are dependent upon a variety of situations related to the patient including their level of consciousness as well as the evident signs, symptoms, and emotional status, among others.

Initial presentation

Some patients may be brought to the hospital by family or emergency medical services (EMS) who already suspect a stroke. Other patients may be complaining of a headache or imbalance and have no idea as to what could be causing their condition. In either case, once arriving at the hospital the patient will first be assessed for signs and symptoms in order to establish their current medical status. In cases where a patient is unconscious upon arrival to the hospital, symptoms cannot be determined and the medical team has to rely on available signs as well as any information that can be provided by those who brought the patient to the hospital.

Scaling/Grading

In many cases, the medical team may have an initial suspicion of stroke based simply on a description of the events involving the patient (e.g. slurring words, difficulty remembering, etc.) along with their own experiences with prior, similar patient scenarios. When stroke is suspected, patients may be 'scored' using one or more grading tests that can help determine the likelihood of stroke. By using validated grading scales to assess for possible stroke, medical teams can strengthen their suspicion of stroke – or in some cases 'rule out' stroke – and thereby apply the most appropriate medical care for the patient's condition.

Patients transported by EMS may receive one or more grading scales on the way to the hospital such as the Cincinnati Prehospital Stroke Scale (CPSS), the Face Arm Speech Test (FAST) or the related Balance, Eyes, Face, Arm, Speech, and Time (BE-FAST) test, the Los Angeles Prehospital Stroke Screen (LAPSS), or the Recognition of Stroke in the Emergency Room (ROSIER) test. Each scale assesses a unique set of characteristics regarding the patient's current condition, but all are designed to help the evaluator arrive at a conclusion of 'likely' or 'not likely' regarding the possibility of stroke.

The FAST and CPSS are relatively quick and simple tests to evaluate a patient's facial and arm weakness and any abnormalities with speech[164]. Although these two scales are used by medical professionals such as emergency medical technicians or paramedics, the ease of application of these two tests do allow for use by non-medical professionals as well. The LAPSS and ROSIER scales are more detailed in nature than the FAST or CPSS scales and are therefore better suited for use by medical professionals such as emergency responders (e.g. paramedics)[164]. Furthermore, the design of these two scales may help recognize the possibility that the patient is suffering from something other than stroke[165].

Upon arrival at the hospital, the patient may also be assessed by the medical team using the National Institutes of Health Stroke Scale (NIHSS). This 10-minute assessment was originally designed for use in stroke research but eventually became commonplace in clinical settings for the evaluation of stroke[166,167]. The NIHSS assesses the patient for his or her level of consciousness, ability to perform eye movements, clarity of vision, ability to detect sensations, and ability to perform facial movements, along with speech and language capabilities[168].

Vital Signs

Soon after arriving at the hospital, patients will have their vital signs assessed. The process of obtaining vital signs may occur simultaneously with other events such as scoring or while questioning the patient or family members. Common vital signs assessed and/or monitored include heart rate, body temperature, breathing rate, blood pressure, blood saturation, and level of consciousness. Each individual vital sign helps reveal key information regarding the potential for stroke[169]. For example, heart rate and blood pressure provide feedback about how hard the heart is working. Monitoring of body temperature provides insight into the patient's metabolism while breathing rate and oxygen saturation tell how well the lungs are providing oxygen and whether oxygen supplementation may be needed. In addition to the initial patient assessment, vital signs will typically be monitored throughout the patient's time in the hospital.

Patient-specific questions

One of the first steps in diagnosis is to quickly narrow down the possibilities as to why the patient was brought to the hospital. In some cases, the reason may be obvious such as if the patient presents with a dislocated shoulder. Other cases are not so obvious, such as in situations where the patient is complaining of dizziness or if the patient is incoherent or even unconscious. Whereas none of the hospital's medical team was present at the initial scene, they must quickly become educated about the patient's situation. This process involves a series of important questions which serve to provide crucial information such as how long the patient has been experiencing his or her condition and to what degree.

One of the first questions brought up at the hospital will most likely be something along the lines of *'what's going on with the patient?"*. Though this open-ended question might sound a little generic in nature, it is a simple question that if answered appropriately can provide the most information about the patient's current situation. It is vital for the patient or family member to provide as much viable information to the healthcare providers as possible. This includes describing the scenario in which the signs or symptoms were first noted. For example, a patient presenting to the hospital with dizziness could be experiencing a variety of medical conditions. Therefore, an accurate description of the scenario in which the dizziness was first noted can be extremely helpful. Saying *she was just lying on the couch and then said she was very dizzy and didn't know where she was* provides very different suspicions for the medical team than *she fell off a stepstool and banged her head against the floor. When she got up, she said she was very dizzy and didn't know where she was.* The first description indicates neural dysfunction occurring without any head trauma, which can help lead to a suspicion of stroke or related event. The second scenario suggests neural dysfunction occurring after head trauma, likely leading to a suspicion of concussion or possibly a subdural hematoma. Even a simple but precise response can provide essential information to initiate appropriate medical care for the patient.

Another likely question will be related to how long the patient has been exhibiting their signs or symptoms. Medical professionals asking this question are wanting to compare the patient's current medical status against the length of time he or she has been experiencing symptoms. For example, lingering dizziness could be caused by conditions ranging from an inner-ear disorder to dehydration to heart attack. If the dizziness has been going on for weeks with no real effect on the patient's ability to perform household chores, it's less likely to be heart-related or neural in nature and more likely (though not guaranteed) to be caused by something in the inner ear which can be annoying but not generally life-threatening. However, a patient experiencing loss of balance and an inability to remember her name for the past two hours leads more towards possible brain injury such as concussion or stroke and needs immediate medical attention. Although the patient, family, or friends may not be able to remember the exact length of time that the patient has been exhibiting symptoms, a best-guess estimate will often suffice.

A third question you will likely hear will be along the lines of *"is there any personal or family history we should be aware of?"*. This question seeks to determine whether the patient is experiencing something they (or their relatives) have dealt with prior to their current medical event. In some cases, the patient may be experiencing symptoms from a medical condition that they or a family member have dealt with before. For example, a patient arriving at the hospital with chest pain may have had a mild case of angina three years ago. This information could alert the medical team to be aware of the possibility of a recurrence of angina, but the team will still check for evidence of a possible heart attack. Likewise, a patient currently complaining of stomach pain should inform the medical team of her mother's history of Crohn's disease as it could reveal a possible cause for her stomach pain and prevent unnecessary testing.

Additional questions may be asked, all of which are designed to extract important information. For example, the answer to *what was the patient doing immediately prior to when the symptoms first appeared* could help establish whether the patient was straining or engaged in intense physical effort, either of which can cause a brief increase in blood pressure or increased pressure inside the skull – both capable of causing stroke[170]. Similarly, the question *has there been any change since you first noticed signs or symptoms* attempts to assess whether the patient's status has changed, specifically if they are getting worse or better as time progresses.

There may also be new characteristics about the patient which are only evident to the family or care providers because of their intimate understanding of the patient's personality. Such characteristics may include unusual giddiness or ongoing laughter, or evidence of the patient being unusually reserved or aggressive. Although such situations may be subtle or seem unusual, if they are not a normal part of the patient's personality it should be brought up to the medical team as it could contribute information about the patient's underlying medical condition.

Many more relevant questions may be brought up by the medical team upon the patient's initial entry to the hospital. For a stroke patient, the responses to these questions can play a direct role in subsequent care. Therefore, it is important that the patient and/or family members provide as much information as possible to the hospital staff, always erring on the side of *over-providing* background information rather than not providing enough information.

Functional Assessment

Patient-centered questions serve as a sort of 'feeling out' period to help orient the medical team to the possibility that a stroke has occurred. If provided enough information, the team may move immediately to the process of obtaining diagnostic tests, or they may begin a physical examination. One part of the physical examination includes functional assessments, which are specialized tests performed by the medical team that are designed to determine whether any of the brain's functions are not performing adequately.

Remember from chapter 1 that the brain is effectively the control center of the body. As we have discussed, stroke doesn't damage the brain as a whole unit; rather, stroke damages the brain in specific areas. To help narrow down those areas of the brain which might have experienced damage, functional assessment tests can be used. There are a wealth of functional tests available to the medical team, and each test is intended to reveal information about the degree and possible location of the stroke damage. Functional testing for stroke patients may include:

- moving the fingers or toes
- identifying which toe is being touched
- reading words on a sign
- assessing peripheral vision
- eye tracking (i.e. following someone's finger)
- repeating a series of words
- reaching to touch an object
- assessing memory
- joint range of motion
- assessing muscle strength

If the patient has difficulty in performing one of the tests, suspicion is raised as to the possibility of damage to the associated area of the brain, and later testing may focus on confirming that suspicion. It is important to note, however, that failure to perform well on one of the assessments does *not* automatically indicate that damage has occurred. Other issues may be interfering with the patient's ability to perform the test such as background noise, fatigue, or confusion. If such issues are recognized, it is important to bring them to the attention of the medical team.

Cranial nerve assessment

One quick and simple functional test involves assessing the integrity of the cranial nerves. The cranial nerves consist of 12 pairs of nerves that connect the brainstem and other parts of the brain to sensory organs of the head (eyes, ears, nose) as well as to muscles and organs of the neck and upper chest. Eye movement, balance, taste, swallowing, facial expressions, and even breathing occur in part through signals sent through the cranial nerves. If you've ever tried to follow someone's finger with your eyes as they move it slowly around in front of you, you've had a portion of your cranial nerves assessed. Because the cranial nerves link directly to several key areas of the brain – and because cranial nerves are quite simple to assess – medical professionals are very interested in cranial nerve function after a stroke. The 12 cranial nerves and their function are listed in Table 5.1.

Table 5.1. Cranial nerves and their function.

Nerve #	Name	Function
1	Olfactory	Smell
2	Optic	Vision
3	Oculomotor	Eye movement, Blinking
4	Trochlear	Eye movement
5	Trigeminal	Facial sensation and movement
6	Abducens	Eye movement
7	Facial	Facial movements, Taste
8	Vestibulocochlear	Hearing, Balance
9	Glossopharyngeal	Swallowing, Taste
10	Vagus	Breathing, Digestion, Heart rate
11	Accessory	Shoulder and neck muscle control
12	Hypoglossal	Tongue movment

Cranial nerve assessment provides important information about particular areas of the brain but is not comprehensive in nature. Therefore, additional functional assessments may be used including movement of the toes or ankles, recognition of touch, or strength assessment.

Memory and Cognition

In addition to assessing various body functions, the medical team may also assess the patient's level of memory along with their cognitive ability. Memory and cognition may be incorporated in with the prior assessments or may be conducted independently. For example, if while being asked the earlier question as to 'what happened', a valid response from the patient detailing his or her initial symptoms may satisfy the medical team's concerns regarding the patient's short-term memory or cognition. Other memory-related questions may include *what is your name, who is the president,* or *what month is it*. Cognition-based questions, on the other hand, assess the patient's ability to understand or comprehend. Such questions assessing cognition may include *do you know where you are right now, do you know what happened to you,* or may involve the patient answering basic arithmetic or spelling problems.

Blood work

Depending on the outcome of the initial assessments, blood work may be requested to help lead the medical team towards a diagnosis while also potentially helping to rule out other suspected conditions. Blood work is a simple procedure for the patient in that it only requires a needle stick and about 1 minute of their time. Afterwards, the obtained blood sample is sent off for some very intricate analyses to evaluate various blood components such as enzyme activity, protein concentration, blood sugar levels, etc.

There is no blood test capable of diagnosing stroke. Rather, blood tests are used to look for abnormalities within the blood that indicate something is 'off' within the body. For example, high red blood cell or platelet counts could indicate an issue with the body's clotting factors. Because blood clots can be a cause of stroke, elevated levels of red blood cells or platelets in the blood can indicate an increased possibility for ischemic stroke.

Conversely, very low platelet counts suggest a potential problem with blood clotting, thereby increasing the potential that the patient could have experienced a hemorrhagic stroke or may have difficulty stopping any current bleeding.

Complete Blood Count

The ordering of a complete blood count (CBC) is generally used to gain an overall assessment of the main blood components and also determine certain physical properties of those components. Cells assessed with a CBC test include red blood cells, white blood cells, and platelets. However, additional information can be extracted by assessing the quality of each cell. For example, in assessing red blood cell quality, a CBC can determine:

- **Mean corpuscular volume (MCV):** a measurement of the average red blood cell size
- **Mean corpuscular hemoglobin (MCH):** a measurement of the average amount of hemoglobin inside the red blood cells
- **Mean corpuscular hemoglobin concentration (MCHC)**: a measurement of the hemoglobin concentration
- **Red cell distribution width (RDW):** assessing the variation in the size of red blood cells

White blood cells, which are a vital component of the body's immune system, are also assessed through a traditional CBC. More detailed white blood cell measures can also be ordered to assess for the makeup of basophils, neutrophils, eosinophils, lymphocytes, and monocytes, all of which have independent roles in relating to the immune system.

Platelet counts are also provided in a CBC test. As discussed earlier, platelet number is indicative of the body's ability to clot. Too high of a platelet number on the CBC indicates an increased likelihood for clotting while too low of a number suggests the body is susceptible to ongoing bleeding due to a suppressed clotting process.

Blood chemistry

Whereas the CBC test is focused mainly on red and white blood cells as well as platelets, blood chemistry tests are used to determine the levels of a variety of circulating components within the blood. Examples of what may be assessed via blood chemistry include glucose levels, sodium concentration, or enzymes such as alanine transaminase (ALT). The most common blood chemistry test is known as the 'Chem 7' which is used to assess general overall health by determining circulating levels of seven different metabolic factors within the blood that include:

- Blood urea nitrogen (BUN)
- Carbon dioxide (CO2)
- Creatinine
- Serum chloride
- Serum glucose
- Serum potassium
- Serum sodium

These factors represent a variety of metabolic processes within the body and provide essential information as to kidney, pancreas, and lung function. Although abnormal blood chemistry results are not evidence of a stroke itself, those results can provide guidance toward stroke treatment. For example, elevated sodium or glucose levels may indicate the need for nutritional considerations in addition to any stroke treatment plan so as to prevent any worsening effects during treatment.

A variety of additional blood tests are available including measures that can assess hormone levels or clotting factors as well as determine a patient's susceptibility to clot formation or risk of infection,. Knowing a patient's values for these blood components can play a role in treatment and may help to reduce a patient's risk of recurrent stroke in the future.

Imaging

Perhaps the most vital tests used in the diagnostic process for stroke are those capable of developing images of the patient's brain. Known collectively as 'imaging', the most common imaging tests used for the assessment of stroke are either computerized tomography (CT) scans or magnetic resonance imaging (MRI). Unlike the assessment of signs and symptoms, which is highly subjective based upon the information provided by the patient and/or caregivers, or blood work, which indirectly measures a variety of circulating blood components, imaging provides visual evidence of the patient's medical status and serves as an important asset in the diagnosis of stroke.

Because of the accuracy that imaging provides, there is often a sense of urgency for patients suspected of having stroke to undergo imaging quickly upon arrival to the hospital in order to determine the best immediate treatment[171]. At present, there is no specific indicator as to which imaging test should be used in stroke assessment[171]. Rather, the American Heart Association recommends only that " . . . all patients admitted to the hospital with suspected acute stroke should receive brain imaging evaluation upon arrival to the hospital"[171]. Ultimately, the decision as to which imaging type is used will be based upon the available equipment at the hospital as well as the available staff[172]. Next, let's take a look at each imaging technique in more detail so as to understand how they are used in assessment of the stroke patient.

Computerized Tomography (CT)

Computerized tomography (CT) is considered the most widely used diagnostic tool for stroke, in part due to its relatively low cost, wide availability, and ability to rapidly provide images[173]. In the brain, CT images can show soft tissue abnormalities such as tumors and can also reveal areas of diminished blood flow[174] along with being able to determine the precise amount and location of existing blood that may have leaked from a hemorrhaged area.

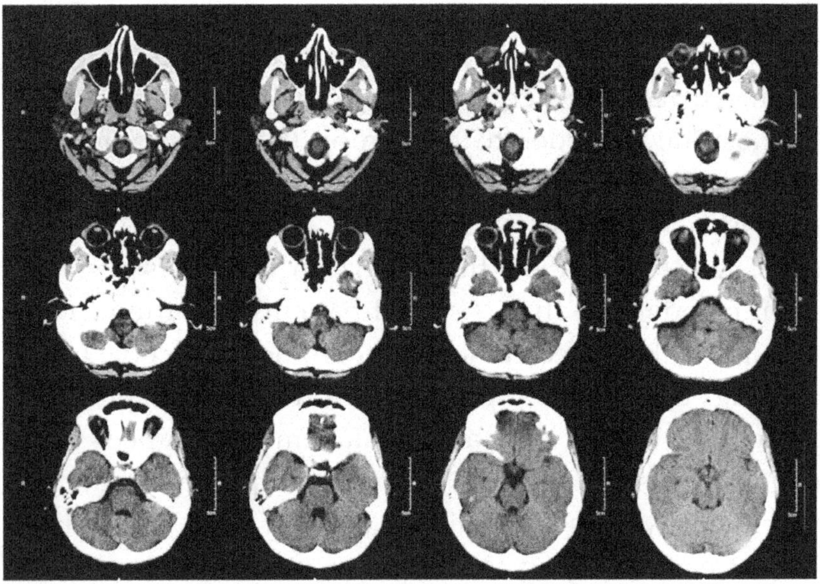

Figure 5.1. CT scans use x-ray technology to develop individual 'slice' images of tissue that can be viewed individually or electronically compiled into a single composite image

A final CT image is developed from multiple X-ray images (called 'slices') that are each taken a very small distance apart (see Figure 5.1). The CT scanner's internal computer then organizes the slices to create a three-dimensional image (called a 'composite') of the patient's brain. Think of a CT scan's individual x-ray slices as slices of bread which, when stacked next to their neighboring bread slices form a loaf. This final loaf can be digitally rotated and examined in detail, and by electronically removing certain bread slices you can see precise details within the loaf's interior.

Although traditional CT is often the first imaging device used for suspected stroke patients, it may not be sensitive enough to detect early ischemic stroke[175]. Therefore, a special dye can be injected intravenously to produce what is known as 'contrast' CT (also known as a CT angiography) to improve the imaging. Contrast CT further enhances the imaged structures and can also reveal the flow of blood through the brain along with being able to identify vessel occlusions, malformations, or tears, including the presence of an aneurysm[176].

Magnetic Resonance Imaging

The other main imaging option in stroke diagnosis is magnetic resonance imaging (MRI). Whereas CT scans utilize x-rays to develop an image, the MRI involves magnetic fields in conjunction with the application of radio waves. Like CT scans, MRIs build images by compiling multiple slices that can then provide a three-dimensional image of the affected tissues (see Figure 5.2). Because of its technology, MRI can provide more detail than CT scans when imaging soft tissue structures such as the brain[177].

Because its technology continues to improve, the use of MRI has been on the rise over the last couple of decades. For example, between the years 1999 and 2008, MRI scanning of ischemic stroke patients increased from 28% to 66% of patients, with over 90% of those patients receiving both an MRI and CT scan[178]. Still, the equipment costs and staffing requirements associated with MRI make it a less-commonly available option than CT, particularly in rural areas[179].

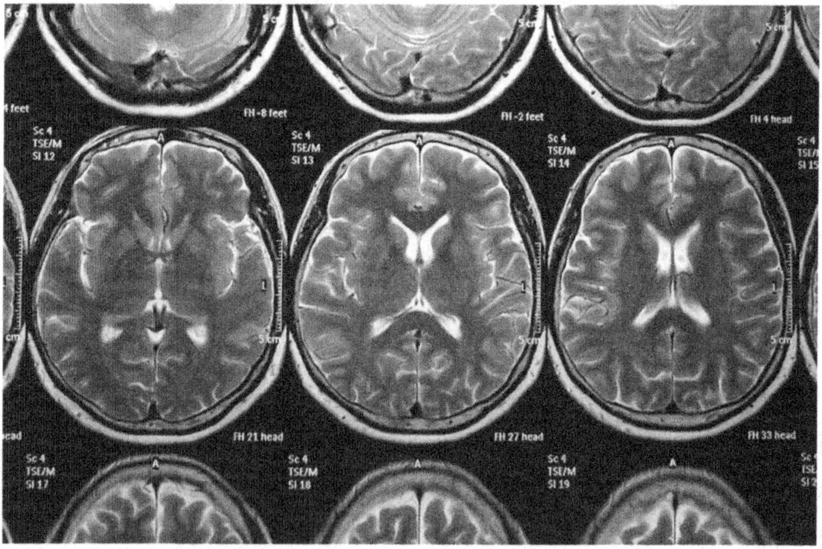

Figure 5.2. Though the images may look similar to CT scans, MRI utilizes different technology and is generally considered superior to CT at identifying stroke

Compared to CT imaging, MRI is considered to have an improved ability to detect acute stroke[180] and has up to five times more precision than CT in detecting both ischemic stroke[180] and small lesions such as those that occur with minor stroke. Furthermore, MRI is reported to be better at recognizing acute ischemic stroke than CT[181]. Perhaps most encouraging is that when using a technique known as diffusion-weighted MRI, the MRI is able to detect damage within minutes of an ischemic stroke's occurrence[176].

Conclusion

Upon arrival at the hospital, a patient suspected to be experiencing a stroke will pass through several stages in the diagnostic process. At each stage, relevant information such as patient history or blood analysis results will dictate the direction taken for the subsequent stage. Diagnostic testing procedures will be used to gain evidence toward the likelihood of stroke while at the same time providing vital information that can help rule-in or rule-out other medical conditions. Imaging can often reveal the presence of cerebral ischemia or hemorrhage, thereby allowing the medical team to arrive at a diagnosis of stroke. As you probably now know, the medical team involved in stroke care involves a wide range of individuals from a variety of medical specialties. In the next chapter we will take a deeper look at the individuals most likely to be involved in the stroke care team, briefly outlining their responsibilities along with their level of training.

Chapter 6 – The stroke care team

During a patient's time in the diagnosis, management, and treatment phases of stroke care, he or she is going to come into contact with a wide variety of medical professionals. Each of these professionals has specialized training in a certain aspect of the stroke care process whether that involves initial management or outpatient rehabilitation. During the early stages of stroke management – when critical procedures are occurring at a frantic pace – it can be difficult for patients and their caregivers to differentiate the roles and responsibilities of each medical team member that enters the patient's room. In this chapter we will look at some of the various individuals that make up the stroke care team, allowing you to better differentiate between the many healthcare providers that you will come into contact with throughout the phases of stroke care.

As we discussed in the previous chapter, stroke management and treatment differs for each patient and differs between each hospital and rehabilitation facility.

Therefore, you may or may not interact with all team members outlined in this chapter. This may be due to the patient's condition, a facility's available staffing, or because of overlap between specialties that allow multiple tasks to be covered. This can occur in such cases where a nurse might also be a phlebotomist, or perhaps when an attending physician is also a cardiovascular surgeon specializing in stroke care.

Physician Care

Directing the stroke patient's care will most likely occur through a team of physicians who each specialize in a certain field of medicine that is inherent to stroke care. Physicians graduate from medical school and hold either a Doctor of Medicine (MD) or Doctor of Osteopathy degree (DO). After medical school, most all physicians complete a *residency* where they take the foundational knowledge learned in medical school and specialize in an area of medicine such as cardiology, orthopedics, or emergency medicine, among others. Some physicians may have pursued an additional research degree in conjunction with their medical training such as a Doctor of Philosophy (PhD), or may have taken a business-oriented route and pursued a Master's of Business Administration (MBA) or similar advanced degree.

The team of physicians are either tied directly to the decision-making process involved in stroke care or collaborate with the primary medical team to provide specialized care, such as a radiologist who coordinates and reads medical images and reports the results back to the attending physician. At all times, patient care is the priority for each medical team member, so they will often work closely with each other to provide the best care.

Attending physician: Physician responsible for the overall care of a patient

Anesthesiologist: Specializes in anesthesia care before, during, and after surgery as well as the administration of any needed anesthetics such as those to help control pain

Cardiologist: Specializes in treating conditions in the heart and blood vessels

Fellow: A board-certified physician who has completed his or her residency and is seeking specialized training in a particular area of medicine

Neuro-intensivist: Specializes in providing critical care for patients with brain and other neurological disorders

Neurologist: Specializes in the diagnosis, management, and treatment of the brain and nervous system including diseases such as Alzheimer's, epilepsy, migraine, multiple sclerosis, and stroke

Neuroradiologist: Specializes in the use of radioactive substances such as x-rays and computerized tomography (CT) for diagnosing and treating diseases of the nervous system

Neurosurgeon: Specializes in the diagnosis and/or surgical treatment of the nervous system and brain

Physiatrist (Physician Medicine and Rehabilitation): Specializes in non-surgical care for nerve, muscle, and bone disorders with a goal to improve overall functioning

Pulmonologist: Specializes in diagnosis and treatment of lung and other respiratory conditions

Radiologist: Specializes in diagnosing and treating disease and injury through the use of imaging techniques. Such imaging can occur through the use of x-rays, computed tomography (CT), magnetic resonance imaging (MRI), positron emission tomography (PET), or ultrasound, among others

Resident: A graduate of medical school who is seeking additional experience in order to specialize in a particular area of medicine (e.g. dermatology, neurology, etc.)

Vascular neurologist: Often called a 'stroke doctor', this physician specializes in the diagnosis, management, and treatment of brain and spinal cord vascular disease

Vascular surgeon: specializes in the diagnosis and surgical treatment of the vascular system.

Nursing

Nurses involved in stroke care are highly trained specialists who carry out a wide range of functions under the direction of the attending physician. Nurses, like physicians, have a wide variety of specializations and training but do not always attend a residency program as is typical for physicians. Nurses must graduate from a nursing program, after which they choose an employment setting in which to work (e.g. family medicine, surgery, neuro-intensive, etc.) The pathway to achieving the title of 'nurse' has many different options, as discussed next.

Certified Nurse Assistant (CNA): Specializes in assisting nurses and providing basic assistance to patients such as helping them with daily activities the patient may have trouble performing on their own. Requires specific training and achievement of a CNA certificate, though some CNAs may possess a college degree.

Licensed practical nurse: Specializes in providing basic care for patients and work under the supervision of a registered nurse. Requires specialized training and completion of an accredited practical nursing certificate program and passing a licensure exam.

Nurse anesthetist: A registered nurse with specialized training in anesthesia. Requires a nursing degree, graduation from a nurse anesthetist program, and passing of a national certification and state licensure exam.

Nurse practitioner: A nurse with a specialized graduate degree who can provide a higher level of care and services than a registered nurse. Depending on the state in which the nurse practitioner is employed in, he or she may be able to diagnose, prescribe medications, and perform certain procedures.

Registered nurse: Specializes in patient care and works under the direction of a physician. RNs hold a state license in nursing and have completed either a two-year or four-year degree in addition to passing a national licensing exam.

In-hospital patient care:

Dietitian: Specializes in planning and coordinating nutritional needs for patients. Requires at least a four-year degree and completion of a dietetic internship.

Case manager: A staff member who functions to facilitate communication between medical professionals, hospital staff, family members and caregivers, and community agencies to ensure any disruptions in the various care processes are minimized.

Lab work / Phlebotomist: Specializes in drawing blood and preparing samples for further processing in a laboratory. Requires at least a high school diploma, completion of a specialized training program, and passing of a state licensure or certification exam.

Physician assistant: Specializes in an area of medicine and serves as an extension of the physician. Requires at least a bachelor's degree along with graduating from a physician assistant school and passing both a certification and state licensure examination.

Social worker: Specializes in medical crisis care and counseling along with coordinating resources for patients and families. Requires a bachelor's degree and passing of a state licensure exam, though many social workers achieve a master's degree.

Specialized Medical Technician: often referred to as 'techs', these individuals provide skills in specialized areas as requested by the medical team. Examples may include ultrasound technician, pharmacy technician, or electrocardiogram technician who are each trained in and responsible for performing a specific skill such as obtaining an ultrasonic image. Most technician positions require at least a high school diploma and may require a specialized certification in their applicable skill.

Therapy

As soon as the stroke patient is able, he or she will begin what may be a long road to recovery. Post-stroke care is not a 'sit and wait' type of plan; rather, it can require somewhat intense rehabilitation in order to return the body to as much of a pre-stroke level as possible. Depending on factors such as the patient's age, the degree of damage, or the location of the stroke, rehabilitation may occur over several months or may be ongoing for the remainder of the patient's life. The rehabilitation team works with each other and with the patient's primary physician to improve the patient's capabilities to a point that he or she can potentially achieve some degree of independence.

Neuropsychologist: Specializes in assessment and possible intervention of psychological issues related to normal and/or abnormal functioning of the central nervous system. Typically requires at least a doctoral degree in psychology and subsequent internship specializing in neural psychology

Occupational therapist: Specializes in improving functional abilities, typically focusing on upper-body movements that involve shoulder, arm, wrist, and finger motions. Requires at least a bachelor's degree and graduation from an occupational therapy program along with passing a certification and state licensure examination.

Physical therapist: Specializes primarily in improving functional strength, balance, and coordination to improve the patient's ability to perform daily activities. Requires at least a bachelor's degree and graduation from a physical therapy program, though many therapists hold a doctor of physical therapy (DPT) degree. Also requires passing a certification and state licensure examination.

Physical therapy assistant: Specializes in assisting with rehabilitation under the supervision of a physical therapist. Requires graduation from a physical therapy assistant program and if required by the state, passing a certification and state licensure examination.

Rehabilitation psychologist: Specializes in assessing the cognitive, emotional, and behavioral issues that can be impairments to the patient's ability to return to a functional life. Requires a doctorate degree in an area of psychology along with specialized post-doctoral training.

Speech-language pathologist: Specializes in the diagnosis, treatment, and rehabilitation of speech, language, and swallowing disorders. Requires graduation from a speech-language pathology program and passing a certification and state licensure examination.

Conclusion

The stroke care team is an intertwined group of highly trained individuals with the collective goal of minimizing stroke damage and eventually returning the stroke patient to their highest level of functionality. In the early stages of stroke care, an array of medical professionals interact with the patient which can make it difficult for patients and caretakers to separate the various roles and responsibilities shared among these medical team members. As outlined in this chapter, the stroke care team encompasses a broad range of individuals of various levels of training across a variety of specialties. In the next chapter, we will step into the management stage of stroke which begins once a diagnosis has been made. At the management stage, stroke care turns from recognizing the patient's condition towards a goal of minimizing further complications and helping the patient begin the road to recovery.

Chapter 7 – Stroke management

Upon a diagnosis of stroke, the immediate next steps are to develop a plan of care that focuses on treatments which will minimize any additional damage and allow the patient to begin to heal. The plan of care at this stage consists of a variety of interventions tailored to the patient's individual situation and may involve anti-coagulants, medication, or even surgery in some cases. Even though the stroke may have happened hours or even days prior, the sooner that interventions can be applied, the more likely that subsequent damage to the brain can be averted.

Minimizing the length of time between the stroke's occurrence and the initiation of treatment is essential. This can be illustrated by evidence indicating that for every hour an ischemic stroke patient goes without treatment, their life expectancy is reduced by 3.6 years[182, 183]. In fact, *every minute* that a stroke patient goes without treatment, an estimated 1.8 million neurons are lost[172]. For patients who suffer an ischemic large-vessel stroke, it is estimated that up to 120 million neurons – and around 830 billion synapses – are permanently lost for each hour that treatment is delayed. This equates to a loss of approximately 447 miles of neural pathways in one stroke patient's brain – *per hour!*

In this chapter, we will discuss some of the techniques used to manage stroke after diagnosis and also outline some of the more common treatments used in the initial stages of post-stroke care and recovery. In reading this chapter, remember that there are a wealth of options available for both the management and treatment of stroke. Your own experiences may differ from what is outlined in this chapter, and it is important to emphasize that the content is written to help you understand some of the aspects used in stroke management and care – not to serve as a guide for stroke treatments or care options. Each stroke is an individual and unique experience for every patient, and the management and care of stroke as determined by the stroke team will be as individual as the patient.

Initial stroke management

Ischemic stroke initial treatment

With ischemic stroke, the priority focuses on limiting additional damage to the brain by attempting to get oxygen flowing again to the occluded area as soon as possible. To do this, tissue plasminogen activator (tPA), or 'alteplase', is commonly used for eligible patients. Considered a *thrombolytic* (i.e. clot-dissolving) drug, tPA is the only drug currently approved by the Food and Drug Administration for the immediate care of ischemic stroke and works at a molecular level by increasing the activity of enzymes responsible for dissolving clots[184].

Delivered as an infusion (i.e. slow release into the bloodstream), tPA therapy must be started within 3 hours – or in some cases up to 4½ hours[185] – after stroke symptoms are first recognized. After 4.5 hours post-stroke, the risk for a condition known as *hemorrhagic transformation* increases and can result in disruption to blood vessels within the brain and cause subsequent bleeding[186]. Such a strict time window for the use of tPA is why prompt transport of the stroke patient to the hospital is essential, since if there are delays due to issues like misinterpreting or ignoring a patient's initial symptoms, tPA use becomes less likely if the allowable time frame for its administration has been exceeded.

As an immediate treatment option, tPA has its limitations. For one, the relatively short window in which tPA can be applied after initiation of symptoms – not after arrival at the hospital – limits the number of eligible patients who can receive it. In fact, very few stroke patients actually receive tPA administration after reaching the hospital[187]. Of those who do receive tPA, only about 15% make a complete recovery while approximately 3% experience intracranial hemorrhage[188].

In cases where the stroke patient does not make it to the hospital within a time frame capable for using tPA, or in cases where tPA use may not be viable, another available treatment option is *thrombectomy.* With thrombectomy, manual removal of the blood clot or thrombus occurs using a guidewire inserted through a vein in an area such as the groin. Once reaching the appropriate area, the thrombus is removed through aspiration (i.e. 'suction') or the use of retrievable stents[189].

Recent evidence indicates thrombectomy has improved effectiveness for clot removal compared to thrombolytic medications like tPA[190], particularly in patients with large-vessel occlusion[191]. Furthermore, thrombectomy can be utilized up to 24 hours after the onset of symptoms, allowing it a much longer window for use than thrombolytics[192]. Thrombectomy also has the advantage of successful long-term outcomes in patients with acute ischemic stroke, including both improved functional independence and an improved quality of life[191].

Hemorrhagic stroke initial treatment

With the aforementioned ischemic stroke, the focus is largely on removal of the clot as soon as possible in order to restore blood to the area. With hemorrhagic stroke, bleeding within the brain has occurred that must be stopped as soon as possible in order to restore adequate flow of oxygenated blood to the downstream neurons. Thus, stopping any active bleeding and addressing any blood which has pooled within the skull cavity are primary goals in the treatment of hemorrhagic stroke.

Most hemorrhagic strokes occur in response to a surge in blood pressure such as can occur while the patient is engaged in activity[170]. Because of the risk for active bleeding into the brain with hemorrhagic stroke, immediate management of the patient's blood pressure is critical. Therefore, one of the first management tactics is to attempt to reduce the patient's blood pressure[57]. A target range for blood pressure has been listed as 150/90 mmHg and can often be achieved through the use of medications such as beta-blockers or calcium channel blockers[137]. While reducing blood pressure is important, a challenge for the medical team is to reduce blood pressure enough to minimize any further pooling of blood within the brain while also maintaining blood pressure at a level capable of supplying blood to the brain[57]. Along with the use of medication, the patient's bed angle may be raised in order to help reduce pressure within the skull[137].

In addition to monitoring blood pressure, the stroke team will also be paying close attention to intracranial pressure and neural function in order to ensure that the patient's neurological function does not diminish over time[57]. Patients will also be monitored for seizures, which occur in approximately ~7% of ICH patients[193].

Whereas there is likely active or very recent bleeding into the brain with hemorrhagic stroke, immediate treatment may incorporate clotting therapy to stop any further bleeding[102] from occurring. Clotting therapy can include the administration of medications such as vitamin K or prothrombin complex concentrates which aid in clot formation[102].

If a significant amount of blood has pooled within the skull cavity due to hemorrhagic shock, there is a risk that the resulting pressure could compress the brain and have life-threatening consequences if not addressed immediately. For those hemorrhagic patients showing signs of neurological deterioration – which may be due to intracranial pooling of blood – immediate surgery is warranted[194]. Surgical techniques to reduce the pressure include the invasive craniotomy or craniectomy techniques[195] as well as less-invasive aspiration procedures[196]. Interestingly, hemorrhagic stroke patients do show improved survival rates in response to surgical intervention; however, surgical interventions to reduce intracranial pressure do not appear to be effective in reducing the patient's post-stroke disability level[57].

Conclusion

Ischemic and hemorrhagic stroke have unique causes and therefore require different management techniques in the minutes and hours after diagnosis. Ischemic stroke management focuses on clot removal –

typically through the use of medication – although surgical intervention is also available. Hemorrhagic stroke management aims to first stop active bleeding, then address complications from that bleeding such as relieving any pressure within the skull that may be caused by the pooling of blood. Upon stabilization and subsequent improvement of the patient's condition, attention turns towards rehabilitation in order to maximize the patient's ability to regain as much bodily function as possible. In the next chapter we will move beyond stroke's initial management and turn our focus toward the rehabilitation phase, taking a look at some of the goals and techniques involved in the processes used to help the patient along their path to recovery.

Chapter 8 – Stroke rehabilitation

Once a stroke patient has been stabilized and there are no real suspicions of additional complications, the rehabilitation phase of stroke care can begin. Unlike the diagnosis and treatment phases – which generally have very defined and focused objectives for the patient – stroke rehabilitation is broader in scope and designed around returning as much of the patient's functional capabilities as possible. This involves assessments of the stroke patient's current abilities, setting goals, designing interventions, and periodic reassessment of the patient's capabilities, all in addition to the patient performing the actual skills and therapies designed to improve aspects such as balance, strength, cognition, etc.

In this chapter we will outline some of the main concepts involved in stroke rehabilitation including the some of the principles of rehabilitation, the different settings in which rehabilitation can occur, and the establishment of patient goals. We will also discuss some of the common rehabilitation techniques used after stroke. In reading through this chapter, it is important to recognize that throughout your own experience with stroke rehabilitation you may or may not encounter some of the techniques and goals discussed in this chapter. What we discuss here may differ from your own rehabilitation experience, but it is important to remember that therapies are designed around the individual and their level of stroke. Therefore, your own situation may require unique interventions as designed by your therapy team.

Initiation of Rehabilitation

It should be expected that all stroke patients are going to need some degree of rehabilitative services, most all of whom will continue rehabilitation outside of the hospital setting. The vast majority of stroke patients experience some degree of motor, cognitive, and/or language complications, many of which can be improved over time with rehabilitation[197]. Combine this with the fact that nearly two-thirds of all stroke survivors and almost 90% of individuals who suffer mild strokes will eventually return to their home[198], and the importance of stroke rehabilitation becomes clear. Furthermore, as Americans continue to grow older, these problems are only going to become more prominent, since by the year 2030 stroke occurrence is expected to increase by 25% in the United States[199].

Post-stroke rehabilitation often begins while the patient is in the hospital and may involve small tasks such as arm or leg movements, balance exercises, or even assisted walking if able. In the body, certain tissues such as muscle can begin to atrophy (i.e. 'break down') in response to prolonged bedrest as often occurs in the days and weeks following stroke. As muscle mass is lost, other functions such as balance or posture – which are dependent upon properly functioning muscles – may begin to suffer as well. Muscle atrophy has been shown to be associated with worse stroke outcomes and occurs in nearly half of stroke survivors[200]; therefore, it is important that rehabilitation is utilized so as to ward off the possibility of muscle atrophy. Rehabilitation that involves muscle activation – such as limb movements or walking activity – is the only effective option for countering muscle atrophy and improving muscle function in stroke patients[201]. Just by performing movements during rehabilitation, a healthy level of physical load, or 'stress', can be applied to the affected muscle. This stress can serve to prevent atrophy and allows the stroke patient to maintain or even increase muscle mass.

While muscles are often the target of stroke rehabilitation, there is more to the rehabilitative process than movement-based activities. Deficits in sensation, speech, language comprehension, swallowing, memory, or even bowel and bladder issues may occur after stroke, highlighting the fact that stroke rehabilitation can involve a wide range of specialties and applications[202]. Patients can expect a thorough evaluation process throughout their stroke diagnosis and management phases which will recognize functional deficits that can be targeted during rehabilitation. These deficits will be different for each patient and will require a highly customized rehabilitation plan.

As mentioned, it is important to start post-stroke rehabilitation as soon as the patient is able. Immediately after stroke, evidence indicates that the most favorable improvement has the opportunity to occur in the first few weeks and months after stroke[203]. Patients who suffer a mild to moderate stroke often see the majority of their recovery success within the first seven weeks post-stroke, while patients suffering severe stroke should expect to see most of their functional gains within 20 weeks[204]. In terms of motor improvements, patients commonly experience the most recovery within the first 3 months after the stroke occurs[203, 205]. These 'windows' in which rapid improvements in function can occur serve to highlight the importance of starting rehabilitation as soon as the medical team feels that the patient is capable.

It should be emphasized that these recovery windows are specific to when stroke survivors can expect to reach their *peak* return of function – not a 'full' return of function. Therefore, it is possible that after the initial weeks and months of rehabilitation a patient will see a slowing of continued functional improvement, perhaps even experiencing some degree of lingering disability.

For example, as many as 30% of stroke survivors report ongoing complications even four years after stroke, in areas including difficulty with independence, trouble engaging with others, or inadequately fulfilling societal roles such as those of being a husband, daughter, or parent[206]. Furthermore, up to one quarter of all stroke survivors may fail to regain the ability to walk without physical assistance[207] and even among those that do regain walking ability, many report difficulty in areas such as walking speed or endurance, as well as trouble navigating obstacles such as stairs or curbs[197].

The possibility for these lingering effects underscores the fact that rehabilitation may extend indefinitely after stroke. The total timeframe for a patient's rehabilitation can certainly depend on the patient's degree of functional deficits but can also be impacted by other factors including the severity and location of the stroke, the patient's age, pre-stroke health status, personal motivation, or the quality of rehabilitative services provided[197, 208]. Still, for many patients a significant improvement after stroke may not be possible due to the degree of brain injury from the stroke. In those patients, rehabilitation can continue for years after stroke, well beyond the 'traditional' stroke rehabilitation timeline. Still, the overall goal remains to rehabilitate the patient and return as much functionality as possible even though a return to pre-stroke levels may not be likely.

Principles of stroke rehabilitation

Functionality and independence are characteristics used to measure the patient's ability to engage in reasonable activities of daily living and also increase the patient's mobility after stroke[197]. Once a stroke has occurred and deficiencies have been identified, these characteristics can be strengthened through rehabilitation techniques designed to improve existing pathways while introducing adaptive methods that can accommodate for the damaged ones. Such adaptations can include learning how to perform a task in new ways, using the opposite hand to write, or incorporating the use of assistive devices to help the patient walk. In fact, that is one of the key goals of post-stroke rehabilitation – to teach the patient new ways to compensate for any remaining disabilities. For example, one might need to learn how to bathe, or get dressed using only one hand, or learn how to communicate effectively with assistive devices if the patient's ability to use language has been affected[208].

Several principles have been developed which provide guidance for focused rehabilitation and maximize the likelihood of favorable patient outcomes and recovery including goal setting, multidisciplinary team approach, task-specific training, and intensity. While multiple variations of stroke rehabilitation principles have been developed, we will next focus on outlining the most commonly discussed principles.

Goal Setting

Recovery from stroke is not a 'wait and see' approach; rather, it is a calculated process based upon the patient's current situation and matched against their potential for recovery capabilities. While it may seem as though rehabilitation consists of having the patient perform repetitive tasks, as we will see shortly there is a purpose in doing so, even though at times rehabilitation can seem tedious and even boring. One of the most important components early in the rehabilitation process is the setting of goals. Goals serve as markers of progress, whether that marker is embedded within a rehabilitation timeline or an indicator of the end of rehabilitation. For example, a stroke patient's goal might involve being able to spread his or her fingers one month after stroke. Reaching such a goal would be just one marker within the patient's overall rehabilitative timeline. Similarly, a goal for a different stroke patient may involve being able to walk unaided. Reaching such a goal may signal the end of that patient's need for rehabilitation, after which the patient is released from care and considered able to function independently.

Goal setting has long been identified as a key part of solving complex problems, and the multifaceted reach of stroke can certainly qualify it as a complex problem. Goals are typically set by the stroke care team and should consider input from the patient and/or their caretakers[209]. Goals for the patient should be specific, measurable, and time-dependent in nature so that they can be periodically assessed for effectiveness[210]. For example, stroke care team members are often focused on clinical-type goals such as "patient achieved grip strength of 10lbs". Patients, on the other hand are more interested in practical goals such as "I want to be able to pick up my granddaughter". Research has shown that when patients are engaged in the goal-setting process and able to provide input, their confidence is improved and their personal motivation and overall satisfaction with rehabilitation is improved[211]. This increased enthusiasm can undoubtedly benefit the rehabilitation team since an enthusiastic patient can serve to enhance the stroke recovery process[212].

Multidisciplinary team approach

As we discussed in a prior chapter, rehabilitation after stroke involves a variety of healthcare professionals including the physicians who oversee the rehabilitation program as well as therapists, nurses, and technicians. While the goal for all members of the healthcare team is to return the patient to as much functionality and independence as possible[213], the methods used to achieve this goal can vary specific to the type, duration, frequency, and intensity of the rehabilitation. Still, the research is clear that stroke outcomes are improved when a patient is treated by a variety of professionals[214], thought to be due in part to multiple factors including decisions being more patient-focused, increased staff satisfaction, and an improved effectiveness of resources[215].

Task-specific training

Another key principle of stroke rehabilitation is that it should be geared towards addressing goals specific to the patient, a process known as *task-specific training*. Task-specific training involves repetitive practice of a movement or skill (e.g. grabbing an object) that is matched to the intended goal[216]. The medical team will work to design rehabilitation tasks that address existing functional deficits, all designed to work towards the established goals. These tasks may include the use of milestones placed along the patient's recovery timeline that can be used to assess the patient's progress towards reaching those goals. If the rehabilitation team feels that the patient is not progressing adequately, it may require an adjustment to the original goals or a re-evaluation of the rehabilitation tasks being implemented.

Although patients have a variety of tools, exercises, and protocols available to them during rehabilitation, research has consistently shown that the most important approach for task-specific training involves carefully guided, well-focused, repetition[208]. Specifically, repetition-based activity during rehabilitation that uses challenging, progressive, and skill-based activities has been shown to lead to improved skill acquisition[217], likely through a sort of 'brain reorganization' that is thought to shuffle neural organization to make up for those connections damaged after stroke. Therefore, in trying to maximize the re-gaining of movement-based skills it is important that patients involved in task-specific training do not simply 'go through the motions' but rather focus on quality repetitions when performing rehabilitation activities.

Intensity

Along with repetitive practice, evidence indicates that after the acute phase of stroke has passed, intensive rehabilitation produces better outcomes[218], particularly in the sub-acute phase (discussed next) of rehabilitation[219]. In contrast to the benefits provided by intensive rehabilitation, most stroke patients prefer to spend their rehabilitation time being sedentary[220]. In fact, many stroke rehabilitation therapists are hesitant to engage the patient in an intense rehabilitation session, preferring instead to focus on quality performance rather than intense repetition[221]. In light of this, patients and caregivers should discuss with their stroke care team which approach would be best for the individual patient's situation.

Alongside intensity, rehabilitation frequency and duration have been investigated. Frequency, or 'how often' rehabilitation occurs, does not have as strong of evidence for improving stroke outcomes as does intensity. Similarly, stroke rehabilitation outcomes are not well-established regarding rehabilitation duration, which consists of the length of time spent in each rehabilitation session. Based on the lack of strong evidence, at present there remains no established standard as to the duration or frequency of rehabilitation. Evidence does, however, indicate that therapy amounts have been increasing over the past decade with no real detriments to patient outcomes[203].

Rehabilitation phases

Stroke rehabilitation has several stages through which a patient can progress on their path to recovery. One grouping of stroke recovery is based upon time points rather than functional achievements and has been outlined as follows[222]:

Hyperacute:	0–24 hours post-stroke
Acute:	1–7 days post-stroke
Early subacute:	7 days to 3 months post-stroke
Late subacute:	3–6 months post-stroke
Chronic:	6 months or more post-stroke

Others have recognized a slightly different set of stages, based more upon the patient's capabilities than on time[197]:

Hyperacute:	1st 24 hours post-stroke

Acute:	1-7 days post-stroke
Subacute:	Upon transfer from acute care
Community-Reintegration:	When discharged home

For most patients, they will experience all of these phases to some degree during the course of their care. Acute care occurs in the hours following the patient's admission to the hospital, and the amount of time spent in acute care largely depends upon the patient's initial stroke severity. Once the patient's condition is stable or begins to improve, they will likely move into post-acute care[223] which may occur in the hospital or in a separate facility. Post-acute care includes the community reintegration stage which involves *re-organization of physical, psychological and social characteristics so that the individual can resume well-readjusted living after incapacitating illness or trauma*[224]. Community reintegration focuses primarily on rehabilitation as well as re-incorporating the patient back into their 'normal' routine while navigating any existing impairments[225].

For those non-acute phases of stroke rehabilitation that are not defined by a timepoint, the decision as to which phase of rehabilitation the patient is in can be based on several factors including the patient's physical capabilities (e.g. strength, balance, etc.), the severity and current status of the stroke, the patient's health insurance coverage, any need to expedite discharge from acute care, or the availability of a post-acute care bed[226, 227]. Along with these and other factors, it is recommended that providers also consult with the patient, family, and/or caregivers prior to moving a patient into post-acute care[228].

Stroke Rehabilitation Settings

Rehabilitation is often classified as either *in-patient* or *out-patient* in nature. In-patient rehabilitation is performed while the stroke patient is required to remain in the hospital for care and can last from days to months depending on stroke severity. With in-patient rehabilitation, the patient will remain under constant care and monitoring in addition to performing some degree of rehabilitation. Out-patient rehabilitation indicates that the patient has been able to achieve some degree of independence and is able to return home, but will likely continue to attend rehabilitation sessions that are located either in their home or at a dedicated rehabilitation facility.

As mentioned earlier, in-patient rehabilitation may begin while the patient is still confined to their hospital room given the evidence indicating that there are benefits to starting rehabilitation as soon as the patient is ready and can tolerate it[229]. These early sessions will likely be shorter and more frequent, and may be initiated as soon as 24 to 48 hours after the stroke[230]. Depending on how the patient progresses and factoring in considerations such as their functional status and/or insurance coverage, the patient will likely have a variety of settings in which they can conduct their rehabilitation.

An in-patient rehabilitation facility (IRF) is designed to provide ongoing supervision and care to stroke survivors who need intensive and ongoing rehabilitation that may last 3 to 5 hours per day. Patients assigned to IRF will remain within the facility, and rehabilitation is provided under the direct supervision of a physician[231]. Patients admitted to an IRF are likely to improve over time, with an expectation of being able to return to society[231]. Stroke patients may also be referred to a skilled nursing facility (SNF) that specializes in providing in-patient rehabilitative techniques. Patients admitted to a SNF may have a difficult recovery or may require onsite nursing care to prevent any loss in the patient's abilities[231]. The amount of time spent in rehabilitation at a SNF is more variable, though patients often receive up to two hours of therapy per day[232].

Those patients allowed to return home after the hospital will receive rehabilitative care either in-home or at a specialized office or clinic. Patients who receive home health care may have limited ability to leave their home setting but generally have some degree of independence and do not require the ongoing supervision common to IRF or skilled-nursing facilities. Other patients may have the option of choosing out-patient therapy like that provided at rehabilitation clinics or offices near the patient's home. These facilities typically have shorter and less-intensive therapy sessions but are required to engage the patient in therapies that are complex enough that they must be performed by a qualified healthcare professional[231].

Neurorehabilitation

For stroke patients, the majority of rehabilitation will be tied in some way to the damage incurred by disruption of blood flow to the brain. The nerves that connect the brain with various tissues in the body remain intact after stroke, but the decision-making areas in the brain may be damaged. As such, the brain's connection to the body remains, but the brain's ability to make certain decisions about the body is impaired. For example, movement of the arm occurs when the brain sends a signal down through specific nerves that trigger muscles to move the arm. With stroke, the neurons in the brain responsible for making the decision to move the arm are damaged even though the nerve(s) along which the signal travels remains intact. In other words, the connection remains, but the decision-making area is damaged.

The goal of neural-based therapy is to help retrain the brain to use a different neural network to accomplish a previously simple task. Doing so takes time, and certainly takes effort from the patient. This is because growth of the axon is the main requirement for an important concept called neuroplasticity (discussed next) and subsequent recovery of the patient's lost functions.

Growth of the axon is a time-consuming process and is dependent upon several physiological changes within the neuron including new synapse formation in the area surrounding the damaged brain tissue[233]. As these synapses begin to reconnect, the patient's neural network begins to reform, which subsequently allows the potential for regaining function to return. At younger ages, this capability for reforming of synapses is high; however, advanced age decreases the brain's plasticity capabilities even in a healthy brain[234]. Consequently, an older individual who has suffered a stroke has to face not only the challenges involved with stroke recovery but also must deal with a diminished capability to reform neural synapses. This diminished capability could explain some of the difficulty in stroke recovery that is experienced by older patients[234].

Neural-based rehabilitation is different than strength-based rehabilitation because the target tissue in this case is responsible for decision-making. In muscle, physical activity that occurs through muscle contraction is the stimulus needed to prevent atrophy and maintain an appropriate degree of muscle mass. As long as the respective part of the brain can function in a way to determine which muscles to contract – and the nerves linking the brain with the muscle remain intact – the muscle can receive its mechanical stress. Neural-based rehabilitation isn't as simple. With stroke, the nerve responsible for sending the signal isn't usually damaged; rather, it's the neural network responsible for decision-making that is affected – and that becomes more complicated.

Neurorehabilitation attempts to 'reorganize' the brain to allow a new area to take over for the damaged area and send a signal along the nerve pathway that still remains. When areas of the brain are damaged after stroke, even though some damage has occurred to a group of neurons, it may be possible to regain some function despite the fact that the original neurons responsible for that function have died. To explain this, we need to address a key concept in neural rehabilitation known as 'plasticity' that deals with how the brain can adapt and recover from stroke.

Neuroplasticity

The term *plastic* can be defined as 'the ability to shape or mold'. Our bodies are in fact highly plastic in that they adapt quite well to any imposed environment. Strength training, for example, is one of the most recognizable ways to show how our body adapts. If we apply resistance to our muscles, they will adapt over time by increasing in size so as to better handle that resistance. Neural networks can adapt as well. Imagine, for example, that you have never stepped onto a basketball court. One day your friend escorts you to the free throw line, hands you a basketball and says "put it through the hoop". What follows will probably be the most awkward set of contortions that has ever resulted in a free throw shot as you try to manipulate your body to heave a ball almost 15 feet forward and 10 feet up in the air with the intention of getting it to pass through the hoop. With time, and through repetition, you soon find that your awkwardness turns to ease as you begin to effortlessly make a few free throws. This change from awkwardness to ease over time is due in part to plasticity.

To account for functions lost after stroke, such as an inability to lift an object with the left hand, one option for stroke patients is to simply compensate and use their opposite hand. Compensation itself does not involve any neural adaptation; rather, the patient simply relies on their functional limb. At times this simple switch in arms is adequate, such as for being able to take a bowl out of a cabinet. But other skills such as buttoning a shirt or walking do not easily allow for compensation since both limbs are required. In such cases, it would be more advantageous if the patient could regain some degree of function in their left hand. In situations where a particular body function has been lost due to stroke, the individual may indeed be able to regain function if the brain can reorganize its neurons through its plasticity capability.

The concept of neural plasticity has been defined as *the ability of the nervous system to change its activity in response to intrinsic or extrinsic stimuli by reorganizing its structure, functions, or connections*[235]. In short, neural plasticity refers to the brain's ability to adapt to a challenge. These challenges can arise from changes within the individual's personal environment, life experiences, or from brain damage itself[236], and can trigger alterations at a molecular level all the way up to restructuring of neural networks[237]. The concept of plasticity itself has itself been around for over 50 years, but only in the past couple of decades has stroke rehabilitation moved to embrace and incorporate the concepts involved in neuronal plasticity[238]. In fact, neuroplasticity has been called one of the most important neurological discoveries of the past century[239]. These days, plasticity is a cornerstone of stroke rehabilitation's key principles, especially given our understanding that repeating activities over and over during rehabilitation helps the brain adapt itself in order to re-gain previously lost functions.

Understanding the principles of neurorehabilitation and the brain's capability for plasticity can help explain a patient's improvement in the weeks and months after stroke. It can also help the patient understand why they are performing specific rehabilitation tasks and why it is important to repeat those tasks over and over again. Changes within the brain take time, and whereas the brain – like many of the body's tissues – operates on a 'use it or lose it' basis, it is important to continue to provide stimulation to the brain through rehabilitation. Next, we will discuss some of the more common techniques used in stroke rehabilitation in order to help you understand the basis and purpose behind rehabilitative techniques.

Rehabilitation techniques

Because the effects of stroke are so broad, it would be difficult for this chapter or even a whole book to outline all of the stroke rehabilitation strategies. Exercises to improve a stroke patient's balance, strength, speech, swallowing, cognition, and even bladder function could encompass several books, and the details of those strategies are well beyond the scope of this book. Even within a specific rehabilitation task – such as working on 'finger dexterity' – there can be many different ways to perform the task and many different techniques to help the patient regain that function, as well as a variety of expected outcomes that can differ by therapist and/or rehabilitation facility. As a result, this section will focus primarily on major rehabilitative concepts, emphasizing the most common strategies used in motor control. As has been discussed prior, your own experiences with stroke rehabilitation techniques will be dependent upon the variables involved in you or your loved one's unique stroke. Therefore, it must be said again that you may or may not encounter the techniques outlined next. The techniques discussed are only a fraction of available rehabilitative options, and there are a wealth of individual exercises and techniques available that may be well-suited for you or your loved one's rehabilitation.

Strength and Range of Motion

The human body is a pretty fascinating organism in that the more you work the body, the stronger it can become. If, on the other hand, you don't stress the body it can become weaker and less able to perform. When it comes to muscle strength, we discussed earlier in this chapter that the body requires you to use your muscles or they may be subjected to atrophy. With atrophy and subsequent diminished strength comes a variety of other consequences such as weakness, difficulty walking or performing activities such as stair climbing, or postural complications. Rehabilitation exercises can help ward off any atrophy and can in many cases improve muscle strength, thereby helping with issues such as balance, posture, and even endurance. Strength is important as it is an essential requirement for normal activities such as lifting objects, walking, or getting out of a chair. Rehabilitation that focuses on strength will likely involve placing a stress on muscles and may occur through activities such as lifting light weights or having the patient perform activities that load the affected muscles, such as getting in and out of a chair.

Range of motion relates to how much normal movement a joint has, and like strength, is important for an individual's daily activities. As we age, range-of motion-naturally decreases, but non-use of a limb can further diminish that limb's normal range- of-motion. Over time, as a joint fails to move through its normal range it can experience 'contracture', a condition that occurs in response to ligaments and tendons tightening and subsequently allowing less movement of a joint. In joints such as the shoulder, diminished range-of-motion can result in an inability to get dressed or reach an object on a shelf. Diminished hip range-of-motion may result in difficulty sitting or standing, or cause issues with physical activity. However, relatively simple rehabilitation can be implemented to prevent any loss of range of motion, and potentially even improve a joint's mobility. Rehabilitation to increase or maintain range-of motion-typically utilizes motion-based activity such as stretching or light exercise to help maintain joint mobility after stroke.

Constraint-induced movement therapy

For patients who experience stroke damage to a limb, it is common – and perhaps expected – that he or she will prioritize use of their functional limb over the limb affected by stroke. Over time, the patient will likely lose strength, muscle mass, and possibly range-of-motion in the damaged limb if he or she continues to favor the uninjured limb. While using the functional limb is certainly understandable and necessary for the patient to perform daily activities, it invites a situation known as 'learned non-use' in which the patient effectively reduces any future likelihood of using the affected limb because they continue to favor the uninjured limb. With your new understanding of plasticity, you can recognize that continuing to use only the functional limb will further ensure that the non-functional limb remains non-functional and will fail to re-build neural connections that were damaged from the stroke. With stroke rehabilitation, the idea is to employ methods that attempt to restore not only function back to the limb but also ensure that it is strong enough to perform activity and can move through a range-of-motion required for that activity. To do so, rehabilitation will be designed to involve the non-functional limb in order to help re-organize neural networks in the brain while also stressing the associated muscles.

Constraint-induced movement therapy (CIMT) focuses on learned non-use (i.e. ongoing preferred used of the functional limb) and forces the patient to use their stroke-affected arm by 'restraining' their functional arm. Restraint can occur by having the patient wear a sling that binds their functional arm against their body, or through the use of a bulky glove on their healthy arm that makes a task difficult to perform, thereby requiring them to use the arm affected by stroke. For those patients showing stroke damage in their upper extremity, CIMT is considered highly effective for improving patient outcomes related to hand function[240], and has particular benefit in improving dexterity[241].

Balance and Ambulation

Balance is often compromised after stroke[242]. Furthermore, ambulation (i.e. walking without assistance) and physical fitness levels have been shown to be very low following a stroke[243]. In the days and weeks after the stroke event it is common for the patient to be either largely confined to a bed or spending a majority of their time off their feet. Maintenance of balance is determined by many factors including sensors in your extremities and joints as well as balance organs within your inner ear. Without constant use of these organs due to continued bedrest – combined with likely atrophy resulting from inactivity – the brain may become less sensitive to balance input which can result in a stroke patient's increased risk for falls[244].

Although balance is required to some degree with activities such as sitting, it is most often involved when standing or walking. Rehabilitation works to strengthen the neural connections responsible for balance, and exercises to enhance balance can occur independently or can be incorporated together with movement-based activities. Examples of balance activities might include standing still on one or two legs, or exercises that require the patient to reach for an object while maintaining their balance[245]. Balance rehabilitation incorporated with movement might include sitting and rising from a chair, assisted or unassisted walking tasks, or treadmill walking that may or may not include body weight support, as discussed next.

Body weight-supported treadmill training

Patients whose stroke has affected their lower body may benefit from body weight-supported treadmill training (BWSTT) which allows patients to work on gait despite being unable to fully support their own weight. Patients engaged in BWSTT walk on a treadmill while being partially supported by a harness (see Figure 8.1).

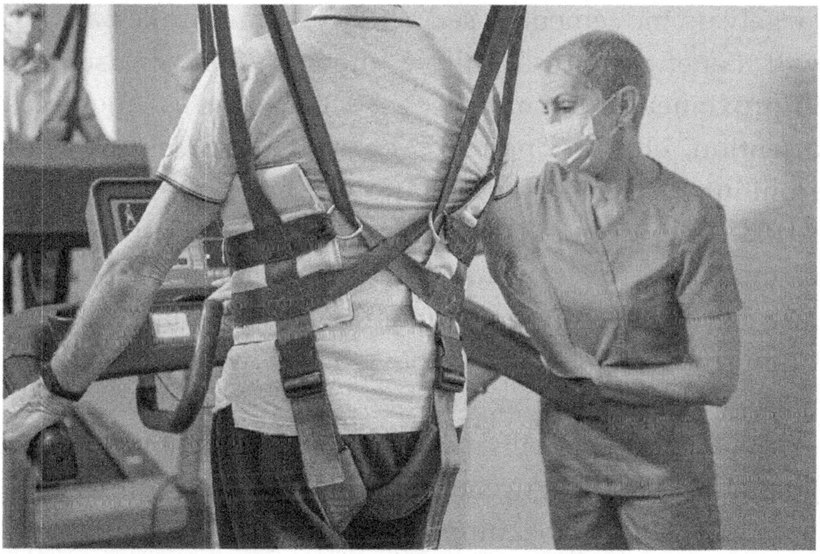

Figure 8.1. The use of a harness in conjunction with treadmill use can be effective at helping patients regain walking capabilities

The harness serves to reduce the patient's risk of falling and takes some of the weight off the patient's legs, thereby allowing them to focus on aspects such as trunk and knee alignment, leg swing, stride length, and walking speed[246]. This in turn allows gait training to begin in the early stages of stroke recovery for affected patients and provides a better opportunity for gait training than does normal walking activity[247].

Cognitive rehabilitation

Along with physical rehabilitation that focuses largely on movement-based activity, some stroke patients will benefit from cognitive therapy that focuses on improvements in mental aspects such as memory, attention, etc. A patient's cognitive capabilities arise from interactions between various areas of the brain, and stroke can disrupt these interactions in a way that ultimately affects characteristics such as attention, memory, or decision making and organizational skills[248]. Cognitive impairment can have a significant effect on a patient's ability to live independently after stroke, even after physical rehabilitation has been successful[249]. The goal for cognitive rehabilitation is to improve the patient's ability to comprehend, answer, and explain information presented to them[250]. However, research indicates that cognitively impaired patients are less likely to participate in stroke rehabilitation activities which can be problematic for ensuring successful outcomes[251].

Cognitive rehabilitation has been described as having two primary principles[252]. First, cognitive rehabilitation emphasizes *restitution,* a principle based on restoring lost function that often uses repeated practice to attempt to restore functions such as attention. The second principle focuses on *compensation,* which attempts to reduce the ways that cognitive impairment can impede functional abilities. For example, common memory-specific rehabilitation techniques include introducing tactics that can help the patient encode, store, and retrieve new information, and may include compensatory techniques to reduce the effects of their memory concerns. Such techniques might involve having the patient incorporate diaries, organizers, and alarms into their daily activities[253]. Cognitive rehabilitation typically consists of tests designed to challenge a patient's memory and cognition. Paper-and-pencil tasks are often the method of choice due to their ease of use and low cost, but the use of computer tasks[254, 255] and virtual reality are becoming more common[248].

Stroke Rehabilitation Success Factors

The National Institutes of Health has outlined several factors that play a key role in ensuring the most favorable outcomes for stroke rehabilitation. While not all of these factors are modifiable, several can be enacted to help the patient have the most favorable rehabilitation opportunity[208]. These factors include:

1) **The degree of damage to the brain**. This is arguably the most important factor as the degree of damage to the brain after stroke determines the level of recovery needed and also establishes the patient's capability for recovery. Patients who have severe damage after a stroke may have very little potential for recovery if their movement, decision-making capability, and/or awareness do not have some degree of function. With a poor foundation due to significant stroke damage, it can be difficult for patients to make significant improvement. Still, improvement is possible but may take longer for those with a higher degree of damage to the brain.
2) **Age**. Older patients tend to have a slower recovery from stroke. Younger patients, including children, often have a higher level of recovery than older individuals, though the degree of recovery even at young ages is largely dependent upon the degree of damage to the brain.
3) **Level of alertness**. Depending on the area of the brain damaged, stroke may suppress an individual's ability to stay alert and focused, which can inhibit their ability to perform certain rehabilitation activities.

4) **Severity of concurrent medical problems**. Patients with multiple medical conditions (i.e. 'comorbidities') or those patients who have medical conditions that could impede rehabilitation (i.e. 'confounders') may require modified activities as a result of those conditions that exist in addition to the stroke.
5) **The intensity of the rehabilitation program**. When rehabilitation techniques are applied to the body, the body tends to favorably adapt. The degree of adaptation can be related to the level of rehabilitation in that increasingly aggressive rehabilitation can provide more favorable results. With stroke patients, the degree of disability from the stroke may require a somewhat relaxed rehabilitation schedule, which can in turn take longer for the body to favorably adapt.
6) **The home environment**. Leaving acute care and returning to an unfavorable living situation can impede progress after a stroke. For example, stroke patients will likely have balance issues; therefore, having clothing or other items on the floor can make it difficult for stroke patients to move about the house. Even small changes such as having proper-height chairs or handrails in the bathroom can allow the patient to progress properly and add to their independence.

7) **Cooperation of family and friends**. This is arguably the most important aspect of outpatient rehabilitation. Stroke patients are often reliant upon friends, family, or caregivers to perform daily tasks. Having a strong support system can be critical in moving the patient towards independence by ensuring a safe environment, knowing when to aid the patient versus allowing them to do activities on their own, driving them to appointments, etc. Rehabilitation from stroke can take months and even years, and maintaining a strong and supportive circle of friends, family, and caregivers can be key to the patient's success.
8) **The work environment**. It may take weeks, months, or even years before a stroke patient can return to their employment. When they do, it is possible that they will need some form of modifications to their work environment. Patients who are able to return to work and have the most support from their employer will have the best chance of a favorable rehabilitation outcome.
9) **Timing of the rehabilitation**. Once the patient is stabilized in the hours after stroke, supervised rehabilitation can often begin. An early start on rehabilitation generally leads to more favorable outcomes in cases where the

patient is able to handle the level of rehabilitation performed.

It is important to reiterate that success in a rehabilitation program is not dependent upon complete adherence to these factors. Rather, these factors highlight barriers that can affect rehabilitation and also help identify opportunities that provide the patient the most favorable outcomes. Therefore, the more closely a patient and their care providers can align with these factors, the more they can maximize the patient's recovery opportunity.

Conclusion

Recovery from stroke can be a long process with improvement rates tied closely to the severity of the stroke itself. Rehabilitation is often recommended to start soon after stroke diagnosis due to evidence indicating that rehabilitation may be most effective during this timeframe, thereby allowing the patient to achieve the most functional gains. Based on the stroke patient's condition, he or she has a variety of options available as to where the rehabilitation can occur including both in-patient and out-patient facilities. With the wide variety of complications from stroke along with the range of stroke severities that can occur, it is possible that the patient may be involved with rehabilitation for months or even years, including both physical and cognitive techniques. Regardless of the underlying type of rehabilitation needed, repetition appears to be the most effective technique and attempts to capitalize on the brain's capability for plasticity in learning new skills. While it can be expected that a patient will make significant progress throughout rehabilitation, there remains an underlying risk that a subsequent stroke could occur. In the next chapter we will discuss some of the interventions used to help reduce the likelihood of a recurrent stroke so that the patient has the capability to continue recovering from their initial stroke.

Chapter 9 – Reducing Future Stroke Risk

Once a stroke has occurred, immediate management and treatment begins. With effective treatment there can be significant or even complete recovery from the stroke. In some cases, however, recovery may not be the end of the patient's interactions with stroke. Nearly one quarter of strokes in the United States are recurrent in nature, in that they are a subsequent stroke that occurs after the patient's initial stroke event[256]. Recurrent strokes can have considerable consequences for the patient, especially those patients who have made substantial recovery after their initial stroke.

Reducing the risk of recurrent stroke is particularly important in light of the fact that people are living longer, thereby lengthening the timeframe in which a recurrent stroke could occur[257]. The estimated risk for stroke recurrence is as high as 16% within the first year and increases around 4% each subsequent year, while the risk of additional disabilities brought on by a recurrent stroke increases by over 50%[256]. Depending on whether the patient's initial stroke was ischemic or hemorrhagic in nature, preventative measures will focus on minimizing the opportunity for a recurrent stroke while also managing the patient's current condition. In this chapter we will discuss several options available for reducing the risk of a stroke recurrence so as to maximize the patient's ability to return as much function as possible after their initial stroke.

Anti-platelet therapy

Patients who initially suffered an ischemic stroke will likely be placed on anti-platelet medication in order to reduce the likelihood of future clot formation. For some patients, low-dose aspirin (e.g. 81-325mg per day) can be effective, and has been shown to reduce the risk of a subsequent stroke by 20% each year[258]. Patients may also be provided a dual-medication therapy such as aspirin with clopidogrel[259].

The risk of anti-platelet therapy is that while on medication the patient is susceptible to extended bleeding since their blood clotting potential is suppressed. Therefore, care must be taken to limit the patient's exposure to risks that could cause unwanted bleeding.

Anti-coagulant therapy

Patients who have suffered an ischemic stroke may not be able to utilize anti-platelet therapy. In such cases, anti-coagulation therapy may be applicable. Instead of affecting platelets like anti-platelet medications do, anti-coagulants work by inhibiting clotting factors that are important for normal clotting activity. Ischemic stroke patients who can benefit from anti-coagulation therapy include patients with a mechanical heart valve, those at risk or suffering from atrial fibrillation, or those patients who have an intra-cardiac thrombus, among others[31].

Surgical Intervention

In some cases, surgical intervention may be warranted for reducing one's risk of future strokes. These surgical techniques may involve the altering of arterial linings (e.g. endarterectomy) or the insertion of stents to widen narrow arteries[260]. Other surgical techniques can involve the repair of anatomical defects (e.g. patent foramen ovale) or artery bypass when necessary[31].

Lifestyle modifications

Lifestyle modifications can be difficult after stroke, particularly because of physical and cognitive difficulties that may linger after the stroke[256]. The most common lifestyle modifications include improving one's diet and physical activity level. After stroke, almost 90% of a patient's time is spent in sedentary activity[261], and even seemingly simple activities such as grooming or bathing can demand almost 75% of the stroke patient's energy supply[262], indicating not only the low activity level characteristic to a stroke patient but also emphasizing their impaired activity capabilities. Therefore, it must be realized that physical activity can be difficult for stroke patients in the days and weeks after stroke. However, physical activity is key to their recovery as exercise can significantly improve several metabolic factors including blood pressure, blood glucose, and insulin values[263]. Current recommendations to reduce future stroke risk include increasing physical activity along with reducing the patient's time spent in sedentary activity, perhaps by increasing their time spent standing and walking if they are able[264].

Dietary recommendations for reducing recurrent stroke risk have traditionally included a reduction of sodium and a switch to the aforementioned Mediterranean-style diet which emphasizes fruits and vegetables, whole grains, low-fat dairy products, poultry, and fish. Such diets have been shown to be effective in lowering cholesterol and blood pressure and can also improve blood glucose utilization[256]. While these diets have been shown to reduce one's overall stroke risk, the research is not clear as to whether implementing a Mediterranean diet is successful at also reducing a patient's recurrent stroke risk[265].

Although diet's effect on stroke recurrence is not well understood, evidence is strong for a recommendation that smoking activity cease after stroke. Unfortunately, the research data is relatively limited in its ability to explain *how* recurrent stroke risk is reduced if a patient stops smoking. It is, however, known that patients who continued smoking after their initial stroke had nearly twice the risk of stroke recurrence compared to nonsmokers[266]. Smoking can increase blood pressure, so avoiding cigarettes can aid in reducing blood pressure which can be particularly beneficial for reducing hemorrhagic stroke recurrence[267]. Furthermore, there is a strong association between the degree of smoking (e.g. 'heavy', 'light', etc.) and stroke risk such that heavy smokers have a higher recurrent stroke risk[266].

Conclusion

Stroke recurrence is an ever-present possibility after the initial stroke event. Still, stroke patients can reduce their risk of suffering a recurrent stroke through a variety of methods that can include medication, surgery, or lifestyle modifications. In the next chapter we will shift our focus from the stroke patient to the caregivers. Caring for a stroke patient can involve significant effort on the part of the caregiver depending largely on the degree of stroke that the patient suffered. Because of the effort required, it is important that caregivers be aware of how stroke care can impact their own lives as well as the life of the stroke patient.

Chapter 10 – Caregivers

In the world of stroke there are patients and there are caregivers. Without question, the majority of attention falls on the stroke patient as their care often requires ongoing attention since they may have lost their ability to perform even basic functions such as those involving movement or speech. To ensure the patient remains safe and comfortable, the caregiver must be attentive to the patient – whether that be during the day or on nights when the patient remains awake and restless. At times, the attention required to care for a stroke patient can place heavy demands on the caregiver from a physical as well as mental aspect, leading to the caregiver potentially needing some degree of attention themselves in order to provide a welcome reprieve from the ongoing demands required of stroke patient care. Like many of the topics covered in this book, the experiences and needs inherent to stroke caregivers can alone fill up several books. Therefore, in this chapter we will attempt to touch on the topic by discussing stroke care from the perspective of the non-medical caregiver, such as that which typically occurs from family or friends. Specifically, we will highlight some of the emotional challenges that caregivers face when providing care for a stroke patient.

The role of the caregiver

Stroke can create immediate and unexpected challenges for not just the patient but also individuals directly involved with the patient. Without question, the highest priority of care and treatment should be focused on the patient; nevertheless, providing care can place significant demands upon the caregiver not only to ensure that the care is performed but also to ensure that other 'life responsibilities' are handled. For example, utilities and vehicles have payment dates that must be met. Work obligations must be rescheduled. Children have activities and school that requires a coordinated transportation schedule. When stroke occurs, all of these situations get disrupted while the patient's initial stroke care is being provided. Depending on the severity of the stroke, some or all of these events may be pushed aside in favor of remaining by the patient's bedside as they fight to recover. Unfortunately, these extraneous events like car payments and work responsibilities don't simply go away. And if left unaddressed, they hold the potential to cause further stress in the near future.

To ensure the patient has a viable life to return back to as they recover, the caregiver may take responsibility. The requirements as a caregiver encompass a broad range of events in their role as a coordinator, rehabilitation facilitator, cook, cleaner, financial specialist, chauffer, insurance specialist, and even fashion designer for the stroke patient – all in addition to the caregiver's responsibilities in their own personal life. For example, the caregiver may be a spouse of advanced age that has their own medical issues to contend with, or who may be the sole income earner or insurance policy holder who must coordinate their own work responsibilities in order to provide income or maintain the medical insurance policy. Or, the stroke patient may have held these roles, some of which may have been their responsibility for decades. All of this can create quite a dynamic shift from processes that may have been in place for years prior to the stroke and which can significantly disrupt what the family has been used to – a further cause of stress for all involved.

Caregivers themselves can experience significant personal change within their lives as the stroke patient progresses through recovery. During the patient's stay in the hospital the caregiver may have some degree of freedom given that the patient is under constant supervision from the medical team. This ongoing supervision may allow the caregiver to leave during the workday to attend their job, or get laundry done, or check on a parent. Once the patient leaves the hospital, however, the patient's condition may have improved, but at the same time the ongoing supervision aspect has been removed. As such, the caregiver may feel a heightened responsibility to remain by the patient's side as a 'just in case' precaution. This in turn can lead to further alterations to the caregiver's schedule such as missed personal appointments, diminished work attendance, distracted attention, or perhaps some degree of unexpected interruptions or personal phone calls at work while trying to ensure the patient is receiving adequate care.

There's no question that caregivers are willing to provide care out of a love for the patient, or even a sense of personal duty that they might desire to fulfil. Perhaps they feel that they will do the best job or they feel the need to 'repay' the patient for all the love and help the patient provided them over the years. Regardless of the reason why they want to be the caregiver, it is important for them to understand that the road to the patient's recovery won't necessarily be easy. And, the higher the level of care needed for the patient, the more demands a caregiver will face. Furthermore, with stroke patients living longer and potentially living for a longer time with some degree of disability[268], it may create extended effort on the part of the care provider.

The burden of providing care

In stroke care, one has to be open and honest in understanding that providing for a stroke patient can impose a *burden* on the caregiver. Yes, it's ok to say it!

The word burden simply means *'load, often heavy in nature'*. There seems to be a stigma that saying "I don't want to burden you" implies that an individual is forced to do something against their will that they don't want to do. This does not have to be the case at all! Burden can be associated with many favorable activities, including transitioning to a new job, getting married, or having a child. For example, a new baby in the house can rank among the most exciting and rewarding times in life; however, without question a new baby can place a burden on the parents that includes new financial responsibilities, altered sleep schedules, doctor visits, and unexpected sicknesses.

The issue of 'burden' becomes clear as a stroke patient care provider. In fact, the term *caregivers burden* was coined to describe the psychological weight or load entrusted to caregivers as a result of taking on the caregiver role[269], and stroke is not immune to this burden. Research has revealed that nearly two in three caregivers report moderate to severe burden in providing stroke care[270], and the ongoing care required for stroke can lead caregivers to restructure their life and alter personal relationships, in turn leading to impacts upon caregivers' physical and psychological health[271]. Survey responses of care providers reveal that in some cases, taking care of the stroke patient 'feels like a full-time job'[271] or that "caring is relentless"[272], with spouse caregivers reporting that they are "working a 24-hour day"[273]. These findings are not in any way meant to indicate that care providers do not enjoy or even accept their role; rather, they are intended to highlight that care providers – along with patients – deal with the impact of stroke.

Despite the reports of burden on care providers, many caregivers embrace the opportunity and truly enjoy being the caregiver. Others may embrace the role of a caregiver but soon realize the challenges involved with maintaining their own responsibilities while still providing care for the stroke patient. After all, the time required of a stroke provider is substantial, at almost 9 hours per day with the patient in the three months following stroke and still 7 hours per day a full year after the stroke's occurrence[274]. Realizing the time commitment required of a stroke care provider is important, as it can be helpful for coordinating care and can also allow the care provider to schedule appropriately. Throughout this chapter we will focus on highlighting some of the most common challenges identified of caregivers and also outline how to reduce the potential impact these challenges can have on the care provider.

Caregiver statistics

Caregivers take on the role of providing comprehensive care to a patient across a variety of matters including financial responsibilities, psychological counseling, grooming, rehabilitation, diet, and many others. Across all medical conditions including stroke, the average caretaker is 49 years old, female, providing care for an older adult, and if living with the patient is providing care for over 40 hours per week[275]. One study reported that the average spousal caregiver is 70 years old, with over 75% of caregivers being women in long-standing relationships of over 40 years[276]. Another study reported that approximately 66% of caregivers were women averaging 63 years of age – though the entire age range was 23–89 years. Around 45% were spouses and 40% were children of the stroke patients while nearly half resided in the same household or the same building as the patient[277]. Yet another study reported that caregivers averaged 63 years of age and approximately 66% were female. Consistently, caregivers appear to be of older age, predominantly female, and are taking care of stroke patients of advanced age. These statistics are important given that older age – especially in the care provider – can be impacted by factors such as fatigue and/or health concerns, which as we will see next is certainly a concern among caregivers.

Life restructuring

Along with the actual medical aspects of stroke, there can be significant time demands placed upon the stroke patient and on the caretaker. For example, conducting rehabilitation, which may involve transporting the patient to and from the rehabilitation facility as well as the time spent it rehabilitation itself, may require an entire afternoon. Bathing, feeding, or simply getting dressed may take many times longer than when the stroke patient was healthy. In such cases, the stroke caregiver must be able to accommodate the time demands of stroke care, and these time demands may or may not fit precisely into the care providers available schedule – particularly given the unexpected occurrence of stroke.

Restructuring within the caregiver's life requires adjustments in order to meet the care needs of the stroke patient while also being able to manage the new roles and responsibilities that the caretaker must handle. Examples of restructuring include adjustments to caregiver work schedules[278] including a reduction in work hours or even halting their job completely[279], changes to living arrangements[273], and modifications to the caregiver's daily routine[278]. Such changes to the caregiver's daily routine include adopting tasks previously performed by the patient such as caring for children[280], management of finances[281], or household responsibilities including cooking and cleaning[282]. Caregivers also report having reduced opportunities for social activities like visiting with friends, a lack of time for exercising or playing sports, or less opportunity for travel[271].

Caregivers and their health

The variety of ways in which stroke can impact a person is immense when you consider the behavioral, memory, physical, and communication-related impairments common to stroke patients. These impairments may each require a unique skill set when providing care for the patient, skills which the care provider may have to learn in a relatively short time. Consequently, the demands of stroke care may place a physical toll on the care providers themselves. Unfortunately, during the process of providing care for a patient, caregivers often neglect their own health[283], with half of medical care providers reporting some degree of decline in their health while providing care[284]. Furthermore, nearly 1 in 6 caregivers report experiencing 14 or more physically unhealthy days in the prior month[284], with 1 in 7 caregivers reporting 14 or more mentally unhealthy days over the same time period. In other words, nearly 20% of caregivers report physical or mental health strain at least every other day as a result of providing stroke care. While this sounds bleak, it must be taken in context. The evidence that stroke care has the potential to be both physically and mentally demanding is not intended to draw attention away from the stroke patient; rather, it should highlight the importance of ensuring caretakers are having their needs met alongside the needs of the patient. Remember – stroke care is individual to the patient, and stroke care providers are individuals as well. Everyone responds differently to their role as a care provider, but some individuals may be more susceptible to the burden that care provision may create.

In situations where the required care becomes long-term in nature, it has been shown that the caregiver is at increased susceptibility to a variety of health-related factors including depression, anxiety, diminished cognitive function and quality of life, and stress, not to mention an increased risk of death[269]. Additionally, stroke care providers are susceptible not only to a greater health risk than the general population but are also at increased risk for poor health in comparison to care providers for other cerebrovascular diseases and diabetes[285]! Next, we will take a look at some of the most common areas of stroke care that can have negative impacts on stroke caretakers. Remember, however, that these topics reflect what is reported in the medical literature and are taken from large batches of data. Therefore, the results are not meant to imply that caring for a stroke survivor is problematic or necessarily burdensome. Rather, these results are meant to provide you information on issues which may arise in your own experience with stroke care, along with how to address these issues to help maintain your health.

Caregiver Stress

Stress is a broad emotion and can be characterized as a reaction to a situation which causes physical, emotional or psychological strain on the caregiver. Because it is such a broad emotion, stress can be expressed in many ways including anger, anxiety, tension, fear, or a variety of these and other descriptors. Despite difficulty in narrowing down a way to quantify stress within stroke care, it is consistently mentioned in the research as a factor inherent to stroke caregivers. In fact, stroke caregivers may report a higher level of stress than stroke patients![286]. This stress comes in part from a 'trifecta' of unexpected situations that stroke can cause, including the caregiver's requirement to learn new skills, the possibility of economic strain, and the physical requirements of taking care of the stroke survivor[286].

The source of stress can fluctuate across care providers. Almost 90% of stroke caregivers experience stress as a part of providing stroke care, while one quarter of caregivers report experiencing 'considerable stress'[287]. Separately, around 98% of stroke caregivers report that at least one event associated with providing care can be "fairly to very stressful"[288]. Some of the biggest sources of stress for a caregiver include dealing with a patient's mood disturbances that often fluctuate between sadness and anxiety, along with memory issues including asking questions repeatedly or having difficulty remembering recent events[289].

Research has revealed that the degree of stress experienced by caregivers may be connected at least in part to certain characteristics of the stroke patient such as the patient's mental health and cognitive function[290] as well as whether the patient is experiencing depression[291]. For example, a patient's level of stress has been shown to be associated with their overall degree of impairment such that lower impairment resulted in lower patient stress levels[286]. Similarly, the level of impairment by the patient – which correlated to patient stress – was also highly correlated with caregiver stress.

Minimizing caregiver stress is important not only because of the potential for causing health issues in the stroke patient but also because it can potentially turn stressful for the stroke survivor and potentially interfere with the stroke survivor's recovery[292, 293]. This is supported by research revealing that stroke patients receiving care from a spouse reported less stress if they had a strong and positive relationship with their spouse[286]. Furthermore, caregivers who had meaningful relationships with the stroke patient reported that providing care brought forth a certain meaningfulness for them and resulted in minimal stress for those caregivers[294]. These findings highlight how a strong caregiver/patient bond can help minimize stress for both the patient and their care provider(s).

Despite stroke being an unexpected event, research indicates that caregivers who are proactive in their preparation, who feel capable of providing assistance in emergency situations, and who take advantage of available resources tend to experience less stress[294]. Conversely, caregivers who were more passive and believed that eventually any problems would 'go away' were more likely to report stress[286]. Given the sudden life changes brought about by stroke, these findings emphasize how important it is that care providers reach out for assistance when needed. In fact, a caregiver's perception of available support can influence their overall level of stress such that those care providers who perceive they have greater support are shown to report less overall stress[295]. This underscores the importance of caregivers taking advantage of their social network as well as gaining access to the many resources available to them in order to minimize as much stress as possible.

Caregiver Fatigue

Fatigue among stroke caregivers is not an uncommon occurrence, especially as the care progresses over time. Caregiver fatigue has been defined as *the extreme physical experience of fatigue by carer(s) or caregivers of a chronically ill or disabled family member as a result of performing caregiving tasks*[275]. The definition is further identified by *the caregiver assuming these caregiving tasks out of a sense of personal duty or responsibility for the ill or disabled family member, and this may be for a prolonged or indeterminate period. The care provided is considered outside the norm of role expectations. Physical fatigue, rather than mental, social, or emotional fatigue, is more pronounced due to the excess physical demand of caregiving. Eventually, caregivers may exhibit physiopsychological symptoms of fatigue, including but not limited to irritability, drowsiness, sleepiness, lack of energy, social isolation, palpitations, tachycardia, and/or extreme exhaustion, which do not easily resolve*. Reports of fatigue are common among caregivers, including the issue of impacted sleep[281]. This fatigue can be both emotional and physical in nature. For example, some caregivers report that sleep-related issues can occur in part due to their feeling a sense of responsibility to wake up periodically to provide care or at least check on the stroke patient at night[296, 297].

While fatigue is not consistent across all stroke care providers, certain tactics have been suggested to help ease or prevent fatigue from occurring. These tactics include spreading out caregiving activities and planning adequate rest, incorporating the use of a diary, avoiding activities or situations that may create fatigue, integrating time for relaxation, or seeking assistance with care when needed[298].

Caregiver Depression

While it is well-known that stroke patients are susceptible to depression, caregivers are also at risk of depressive thoughts when providing stroke care. After 1 year of caring for a stroke victim, 50% of care providers report experiencing emotional problems[197]. In fact, as many as 40% of stroke caregivers may be experiencing some degree of depression[299]. Stroke is an unexpected event, and the research indicates that the unexpectedness of having to provide ongoing care for a stroke patient contributes to caregiver depression due to the caregiver feeling unprepared as well as frustrated and lacking support[300]. Another major factor influencing caregiver depression is a perceived inability to be socially active within the community[301] which can leave the care provider feeling isolated. Treatment for depression can include focused psychological activities including cognitive-behavioral therapy, problem-solving activities, and training focused on improving coping skills[302]. Treatment for depression among care providers is critical, as the stroke patient's quality of life can be affected by a care provider's depression[303].

Along the lines of depression is another emotional consequence that can affect care providers – a loss of connection with the patient, whether that patient is a child, parent, or spouse. Consistently, caregivers report a change in their relationship with the stroke patient[304]. Specific to spousal caregivers, reports of decreased intimacy and feeling that the stroke survivor seems almost like a stranger were noted[273]. As the provision of care extends out over time, caregivers will often internalize their thoughts and personal concerns, choosing to not vocalize or address issues which they feel relevant. Doing so tends to ultimately make caregivers silent patients themselves[305], certainly an issue that should be addressed when providing stroke care.

Caregiver Preparedness

Taking care of a stroke patient can thrust a caregiver into a whole realm of responsibilities for which he or she may have no understanding. Upon release of the patient from the hospital, many caregivers are not fully aware of the scope of their responsibilities in patient care[306]. Tasks such as preparing special diets, administering medication, or coordinating at-home rehabilitation are patient-specific demands on the caregiver's time but don't even include additional duties such as bill payments, laundry, or cleaning that must occur in addition to patient care.

Caring for a stroke patient thrusts a care provider into a supervisory healthcare role, and it is not uncommon for the care provider to feel unprepared and even intimidated at the prospect of being the person responsible for the array of responsibilities inherent to stroke care. Caregiver *preparedness* is a term used to outline how prepared the caregiver feels toward providing various aspects of care to the stroke survivor, and it has been shown that better caregiver preparedness is linked to improved outcomes for caregivers and stroke patients[307]. For example, caregivers who identify as being unprepared to care for a stroke patient are more likely to experience negative physical, mental, and emotional health outcomes[289]. Conversely, caregivers reporting better preparedness also report lower levels of burden and stress as well as mood disturbances[308]. Perhaps most importantly, the stroke patients of better-prepared caregivers have improved recovery and quality of life[309].

Even while the patient is still in the hospital, some care providers report feeling ignored by the patient's stroke care team, which in turn can lead to caregivers feeling as though their questions are not being addressed[310]. This in turn can lead to communication issues with the health care team, along with inadequate information regarding the patient's expected progress and post-hospital care needs.

The positives

While it seems we have focused on the negative in this chapter, the idea was to expose caregivers to the true demands inherent to taking care of a stroke patient. It is interesting to note that in reviewing the medical literature, there are similarly a wealth of studies investigating caregiver experiences related to strain, stress, anxiety, and other related effects, but very little attention devoted to outlining some of the encouraging aspects of stroke patient care.

In this chapter we have largely passed over the many positives that can arise from the role of stroke care provider since there can be so much consequential risk related to caretaker issues such as stress, unpreparedness, etc. However, there are indeed positive aspects of stroke care. We discussed earlier how some caregivers embrace the opportunity and truly enjoy providing care. Others report enhanced communication and improved appreciation of the spouse, along with closer family and friend relationships[271]. Some care providers describe finding a sense of meaning in seeing progress in the stroke patient, along with a sense of feeling appreciated and exhibiting increased self-esteem[311].

It is important to point out that caregiving is not an entirely negative experience. Still, it is important that caregivers are aware of the significant changes brought about by the role of stroke care provider and allow them to prepare for this new aspect of their life. In fact, given the effect that preparedness can have towards outcomes for both the patient and the caregiver, it can be beneficial to assess the caregiver's level of preparedness prior to the stroke patient returning home. Whereas interventions can be implemented – which have been shown to improve caregiver preparedness[312] – both the patient and the stroke caregiver can benefit from the improved awareness needed for quality stroke care.

Conclusion

Stroke can place significant challenges upon the patient as well as on those individuals who provide care for the patient. Recognizing the importance of the caregiver has allowed us to recognize that they must be included in the overall concept of stroke care. While the focus of attention is typically on the stroke patient, it is important that the stroke caregiver advocate for their health and create time to take care of themselves – within their overall care for the stroke patient. As we have seen, stroke caregivers can face significant health risks such as stress, anxiety, and lack a sleep, and if these aspects are not addressed adequately they can result in complications for the caregiver and for the patient. Several factors have been identified as contributing to unfavorable outcomes for stroke care providers, and addressing these factors early may help reduce their risk of occurrence. Caregivers who feel psychologically healthy tend to feel better about providing care for the patient – a key reason that the emotional health of the caregiver must be accounted for in stroke care.

Conclusion

It has been quite a journey as we have progressed through a deeper understanding of stroke care. I hope that this book has been able to increase your awareness of the various aspects of stroke and improved your knowledge regarding its causes, treatment, and care. Take a moment to think back on your understanding of stroke when we started this journey. Has this book improved that understanding in any way? That was the original intent of the book – and I sincerely hope that I have been able to follow through on that intent.

Let's take a look at what all we have learned as we progressed through this book. We have learned how the brain works, and how different areas of the brain control individual aspects of normal human function. We discussed blood flow through the brain as well as consequences that result when that blood flow is interrupted. We outlined both ischemic and hemorrhagic stroke, along with the subtypes of each. We discussed the demographics of who is affected by each type of stroke, and you may have recognized how your own experience with stroke matches with those populations. We detailed the associated risk factors for stroke as well as how to reduce those risk factors. We compared the various stroke mimics, some of which you may have heard discussed during the initial hours after arriving at the hospital. We walked through the diagnostic process for stroke, highlighting the various tests and procedures used to help rule-in stroke as well as rule-out the many mimics. We then reviewed the various stroke care team members to help you recognize the roles of the many individuals you interact with during the early stages of stroke. We then outlined the initial steps in management of stroke, detailing the actions commonly used to stabilize the patient and minimize further damage. Then we looked at the rehabilitation phase of stroke, discussing the various principles designed to maximize a patient's recovery. We then discussed how to reduce the risk of recurrent stroke in order to maximize the patient's recovery potential after their initial stroke. Finally, we switched gears and focused on reviewing aspects related to the stroke caretaker, highlighting the most consequential aspects of stroke care and emphasizing the degree of effort that stroke care can take.

When you sit back and take a look, that is certainly a lot of information that you have digested. The key thing to ask yourself, though, is whether you read through the information or if you *understand* the information. If it's the latter, great! If it's the former and you feel that you have simply read through the information, please – read it again. This book was written to inform you about stroke and allow you to have meaningful conversations with your stroke care team members. By understanding the material, you can have those conversations and involve yourself in productive interactions with the care team. This will help ensure that you or your loved one receives the best care that can be provided.

I'm not naïve to the fact that at times this book became a bit technical in nature. As I wrote, I quickly learned that it was difficult to discuss topics like neuroplasticity without including at least some of the underlying science. If it became too overbearing, I apologize. But understand that my intent was to provide you the foundational information without simply providing you a superficial overview. Neuroplasticity, for example, required detailed information about the neuron in order to provide you a clear insight of neuroplasticity. This required a deeper level of detail than I had expected, but I wanted to leave you with an appreciation for the concepts of neuroplasticity rather than just an ability to define what it is.

At one point early in the book it was discussed just how much research is focused on stroke, such as the fact that there are many research journals devoted purely to stroke research or even specialized areas such as stroke rehabilitation. While this is encouraging to stroke patients, it is also important to note that because of this ongoing research, what you read about stroke one day may be outdated a month later as new research provides additional or more-relevant information. So whereas this book was written to try and consolidate much of the information that exists on stroke, understand that new information is constantly coming out. And that is a great thing, as it means that researchers are working to improve our understanding of stroke which will in turn contribute to improved diagnosis and treatment, perhaps even working towards advancements in stroke prevention as well as an increased rate of patients who make a full recovery.

In closing, I hope that this book has been helpful for you in understanding more about stroke. I know that in working through collecting the information for this book, my own knowledge of stroke has improved immensely, and my respect and admiration for stroke care providers has grown tremendously as well. And as for my mom and her stroke outcomes? I guess we can consider her among the lucky ones as her recovery has been nothing short of remarkable – perhaps eventually even progressing into a 'full recovery'. I can only hope that you see similar progress in yourself or your loved one.

Thank you for joining me in learning more about stroke, and I wish you the best throughout your stroke journey.

References

1 Kimmlingen R. Pioneers of connectome gradients. *Magnetom FLASH*. 2017; **68**: 122-36.
2 Rowe WL. The cosmological argument and the principle of sufficient reason. *Man and World*. 1968; **1**: 278-92.
3 Purves D, Augustine G, Fitzpatrick D, *et al.* Neuroscience 2nd edition. sunderland (ma) sinauer associates. *Types of Eye Movements and Their Functions*. 2001.
4 Ruchalski K, Hathout GM. A medley of midbrain maladies: a brief review of midbrain anatomy and syndromology for radiologists. *Radiology research and practice*. 2012; **2012**.
5 Spengos K, Wohrle J, Tsivgoulis G, Stouraitis G, Vemmos K, Zis V. Bilateral paramedian midbrain infarct: an uncommon variant of the "top of the basilar" syndrome. *Journal of Neurology, Neurosurgery & Psychiatry*. 2005; **76**: 742-43.
6 Caminero F, Cascella M. Neuroanatomy, mesencephalon midbrain. 2019.
7 Tyson PJ, Jones D, Elcock J. *Psychology in social context: Issues and debates*: John Wiley & Sons, 2011.
8 Ghosh P, Sagerström CG. Developing roles for Hox proteins in hindbrain gene regulatory networks. *International Journal of Developmental Biology*. 2018; **62**: 767-74.
9 Schmahmann JD, Guell X, Stoodley CJ, Halko MA. The theory and neuroscience of cerebellar cognition. *Annual review of neuroscience*. 2019; **42**: 337-64.
10 Van Essen DC, Donahue CJ, Glasser MF. Development and evolution of cerebral and cerebellar cortex. *Brain, behavior and evolution*. 2018; **91**: 158-69.
11 Davis S, Gupta N, Samudra M, Javadekar A. A case of frontal lobe syndrome. *Industrial Psychiatry Journal*. 2021; **30**: 360.
12 Javed K, Reddy V, Lui F. Neuroanatomy, cerebral cortex. 2019.

13 Velásquez C, Goméz E, Martino J. Mapping visuospatial and self-motion perception functions in the left parietal lobe. *Neurosurgical Focus*. 2018; **45**: V8.
14 Rehman A, Al Khalili Y. Neuroanatomy, occipital lobe. 2019.
15 Borghesani V, Narvid J, Battistella G, *et al.* "Looks familiar, but I do not know who she is": The role of the anterior right temporal lobe in famous face recognition. *Cortex*. 2019; **115**: 72-85.
16 Gong L, Wang J, Feng L, *et al.* Explicit memory and implicit memory in occipital lobe stroke patients. *Journal of Stroke and Cerebrovascular Diseases*. 2015; **24**: 663-67.
17 Tanaka K. Temporal lobe. 2001.
18 Larson J, Drew KL, Folkow LP, Milton SL, Park TJ. No oxygen? No problem! Intrinsic brain tolerance to hypoxia in vertebrates. *Journal of Experimental Biology*. 2014; **217**: 1024-39.
19 Leach R, Treacher D. Oxygen transport2. Tissue hypoxia. *Bmj*. 1998; **317**: 1370-73.
20 Razaaq A, Abdelelah H. A Short Review: Genetic Risk Factors of Stroke. 2021.
21 Ely W. *Every deep-drawn breath: A critical care doctor on healing, recovery, and transforming medicine in the ICU*: Simon and Schuster, 2022.
22 Ravindran S. QnAs with Mark T. Nelson. *Proceedings of the National Academy of Sciences*. 2020; **117**: 20346-47.
23 Gupta N, Zhao Y-Y, Evans CE. The stimulation of thrombosis by hypoxia. *Thrombosis research*. 2019; **181**: 77-83.
24 Caplan LR, Simon RP, Hassani S. Cerebrovascular disease—stroke. *Neurobiology of Brain Disorders*: Elsevier, 2023; 457-76.
25 Hatano S. Experience from a multicentre stroke register: a preliminary report. *Bulletin of the World Health Organization*. 1976; **54**: 541.
26 Torpy JM, Burke AE, Glass RM. Hemorrhagic stroke. *JAMA*. 2010; **303**: 2312-12.
27 Hosseini H. Stroke and cardiovascular disease among women. *Health*. 2015; **7**: 1847.
28 Saif I. Role of physical therapy on quality of life and level of satisfaction among patients with stroke. *The Healer*

Journal of Physiotherapy and Rehabilitation Sciences. 2022; **2**: 104-09.
29 Owolabi MO, Thrift AG, Mahal A, *et al.* Primary stroke prevention worldwide: translating evidence into action. *The Lancet Public Health*. 2022; **7**: e74-e85.
30 Lyden S, Wold J. Acute treatment of ischemic stroke. *Neurologic Clinics*. 2022; **40**: 17-32.
31 Feske SK. Ischemic stroke. *The American journal of medicine*. 2021; **134**: 1457-64.
32 Albert SJ, Kesselring J. Neurorehabilitation of stroke. *Journal of neurology*. 2012; **259**: 817-32.
33 Moskowitz MA, Lo EH, Iadecola C. The science of stroke: mechanisms in search of treatments. *Neuron*. 2010; **67**: 181-98.
34 Béjot Y, Daubail B, Giroud M. Epidemiology of stroke and transient ischemic attacks: Current knowledge and perspectives. *Revue neurologique*. 2016; **172**: 59-68.
35 Phipps MS, Cronin CA. Management of acute ischemic stroke. *Bmj*. 2020; **368**.
36 Benjamin EJ, Blaha MJ, Chiuve SE, *et al.* Heart disease and stroke statistics—2017 update: a report from the American Heart Association. *circulation*. 2017; **135**: e146-e603.
37 Larsen LP, Biering K, Johnsen SP, Andersen G, Hjollund NH. Self-rated health and return to work after first-time stroke. *Journal of Rehabilitation Medicine*. 2016; **48**: 339-45.
38 Benjamin EJ, Muntner P, Alonso A, *et al.* Heart Disease and Stroke Statistics—2019 Update: A Report From the American Heart Association. *Circulation*. 2019; **139**: e56-e528.
39 site CfDCaPW. Behavioral Risk Factor Surveillance System: annual survey data, 2013.
40 Goldstein LB, Adams R, Becker K, Purberg C, Gorelick P, Hademenos G. ea, Primary Prevention of Ischemic Stroke: A Statement for Healthcare Professionals, the Stroke Council of the American Heart Association. *Stroke*. 2018; **32**.
41 Polotsky HN, Polotsky AJ. Metabolic implications of menopause. *Seminars in reproductive medicine*: © Thieme Medical Publishers, 2010; 426-34.

42 Persky RW, Turtzo LC, McCullough LD. Stroke in women: disparities and outcomes. *Current cardiology reports*. 2010; **12**: 6-13.
43 Barthels D, Das H. Current advances in ischemic stroke research and therapies. *Biochimica et Biophysica Acta (BBA)-Molecular Basis of Disease*. 2020; **1866**: 165260.
44 Prevention CfDCa. Stroke facts, 2020. *Retrieved from Centers for Disease Control and Prevention website: http://www cdc gov/stroke/facts htm*. 2020.
45 Lozano R, Naghavi M, Foreman K, *et al*. Global and regional mortality from 235 causes of death for 20 age groups in 1990 and 2010: a systematic analysis for the Global Burden of Disease Study 2010. *The lancet*. 2012; **380**: 2095-128.
46 Demir A, Eren F. The relationship between serum bilirubin levels and early neurological improvement in patients with acute ischemic stroke treated with intravenous tissue plasminogen activator. *Neurology Asia*. 2022; **27**.
47 Adams HP, Davis P, Leira E, *et al*. Baseline NIH Stroke Scale score strongly predicts outcome after stroke: a report of the Trial of Org 10172 in Acute Stroke Treatment (TOAST). *Neurology*. 1999; **53**: 126-26.
48 Sobiczewski W, Wirtwein M, Trybala E, Gruchala M. Severity of coronary atherosclerosis and stroke incidence in 7-year follow-up. *Journal of Neurology*. 2013; **260**: 1855-58.
49 Choi HW, Navia JA, Kassab GS. Stroke propensity is increased under atrial fibrillation hemodynamics: a simulation study. *PloS one*. 2013; **8**: e73485.
50 Yaghi S, Prabhakaran S, Khatri P, Liebeskind DS. Intracranial atherosclerotic disease: mechanisms and therapeutic implications. *Stroke*. 2019; **50**: 1286-93.
51 Yang W-j, Wong K-s, Chen X-y. Intracranial atherosclerosis: from microscopy to high-resolution magnetic resonance imaging. *Journal of stroke*. 2017; **19**: 249.
52 Yaghi S, Rostanski SK, Boehme AK, *et al*. Imaging parameters and recurrent cerebrovascular events in patients with minor stroke or transient ischemic attack. *JAMA neurology*. 2016; **73**: 572-78.

53 Mendelson SJ, Prabhakaran S. Diagnosis and management of transient ischemic attack and acute ischemic stroke: a review. *Jama*. 2021; **325**: 1088-98.
54 Lioutas V-A, Ivan CS, Himali JJ, *et al.* Incidence of transient ischemic attack and association with long-term risk of stroke. *Jama*. 2021; **325**: 373-81.
55 Amarenco P, Lavallée PC, Labreuche J, *et al.* One-year risk of stroke after transient ischemic attack or minor stroke. *New England Journal of Medicine*. 2016; **374**: 1533-42.
56 An SJ, Kim TJ, Yoon B-W. Epidemiology, risk factors, and clinical features of intracerebral hemorrhage: an update. *Journal of stroke*. 2017; **19**: 3.
57 Montaño A, Hanley DF, Hemphill III JC. Hemorrhagic stroke. *Handbook of clinical neurology*. 2021; **176**: 229-48.
58 Chen S, Zeng L, Hu Z. Progressing haemorrhagic stroke: categories, causes, mechanisms and managements. *Journal of neurology*. 2014; **261**: 2061-78.
59 Sacco RL, Kasner SE, Broderick JP, *et al.* An updated definition of stroke for the 21st century: a statement for healthcare professionals from the American Heart Association/American Stroke Association. *Stroke*. 2013; **44**: 2064-89.
60 Van Asch CJ, Luitse MJ, Rinkel GJ, van der Tweel I, Algra A, Klijn CJ. Incidence, case fatality, and functional outcome of intracerebral haemorrhage over time, according to age, sex, and ethnic origin: a systematic review and meta-analysis. *The Lancet Neurology*. 2010; **9**: 167-76.
61 McGurgan IJ, Ziai WC, Werring DJ, Salman RA-S, Parry-Jones AR. Acute intracerebral haemorrhage: diagnosis and management. *Practical Neurology*. 2021; **21**: 128-36.
62 Adeoye O, Broderick JP. Advances in the management of intracerebral hemorrhage. *Nature Reviews Neurology*. 2010; **6**: 593-601.
63 Ziai WC, Carhuapoma JR. Intracerebral hemorrhage. *Continuum: Lifelong Learning in Neurology*. 2018; **24**: 1603-22.
64 Fisher CM. Pathological observations in hypertensive cerebral hemorrhage. *Journal of Neuropathology & Experimental Neurology*. 1971; **30**: 536-50.

65 Barks A, Behbahani M, Alqadi MM, *et al.* A new scoring system for prediction of underlying vascular pathology in patients with Intracerebral hemorrhage: the modified secondary intracerebral hemorrhage score. *World Neurosurgery*. 2020; **142**: e126-e32.
66 Block F, Dafotakis M. Cerebral amyloid angiopathy in stroke medicine. *Deutsches Ärzteblatt International*. 2017; **114**: 37.
67 Foulkes MA, Wolf PA, Price TR, Mohr J, Hier DB. The Stroke Data Bank: design, methods, and baseline characteristics. *Stroke*. 1988; **19**: 547-54.
68 Qureshi AI, Tuhrim S, Broderick JP, Batjer HH, Hondo H, Hanley DF. Spontaneous intracerebral hemorrhage. *New England Journal of Medicine*. 2001; **344**: 1450-60.
69 Romero JM, Rosand J. Hemorrhagic cerebrovascular disease. *Handbook of Clinical Neurology*. 2016; **135**: 351-64.
70 Qureshi AI, Mendelow AD, Hanley DF. Intracerebral haemorrhage. *The Lancet*. 2009; **373**: 1632-44.
71 Rincon F, Mayer SA. The epidemiology of intracerebral hemorrhage in the United States from 1979 to 2008. *Neurocritical Care*. 2013; **19**: 95-102.
72 Krishnamurthi RV, Moran AE, Forouzanfar MH, *et al.* The global burden of hemorrhagic stroke: a summary of findings from the GBD 2010 study. *Global heart*. 2014; **9**: 101-06.
73 Hong K-S, Bang OY, Kang D-W, *et al.* Stroke statistics in Korea: part I. Epidemiology and risk factors: a report from the korean stroke society and clinical research center for stroke. *Journal of stroke*. 2013; **15**: 2.
74 Stein M, Misselwitz B, Hamann GF, Scharbrodt W, Schummer DI, Oertel MF. Intracerebral hemorrhage in the very old: future demographic trends of an aging population. *Stroke*. 2012; **43**: 1126-28.
75 Jolink WM, Klijn CJ, Brouwers PJ, Kappelle LJ, Vaartjes I. Time trends in incidence, case fatality, and mortality of intracerebral hemorrhage. *Neurology*. 2015; **85**: 1318-24.
76 Matsuda M, Watanabe K, Saito A, Matsumura K-i, Ichikawa M. Circumstances, activities, and events

precipitating aneurysmal subarachnoid hemorrhage. *Journal of Stroke and Cerebrovascular Diseases*. 2007; **16**: 25-29.
77 Lawton MT, Vates GE. Subarachnoid hemorrhage. *New England Journal of Medicine*. 2017; **377**: 257-66.
78 Leira R, Castellanos M, Álvarez-Sabín J, *et al.* Headache in cerebral hemorrhage is associated with inflammatory markers and higher residual cavity. *Headache: The Journal of Head and Face Pain*. 2005; **45**: 1236-43.
79 Stalons M, Priemer DS, Knollmann-Ritschel BE. Educational Case: Cranial hemorrhage and traumatic brain injury. *Academic Pathology*. 2022; **9**.
80 Polmear A. Sentinel headaches in aneurysmal subarachnoid haemorrhage: what is the true incidence? A systematic review. *Cephalalgia*. 2003; **23**: 935-41.
81 Edlow JA, Panagos PD, Godwin SA, Thomas TL, Decker WW. American College of Emergency P. Clinical policy: critical issues in the evaluation and management of adult patients presenting to the emergency department with acute headache. *Ann Emerg Med*. 2008; **52**: 407-36.
82 Kowalski RG, Claassen J, Kreiter KT, *et al.* Initial misdiagnosis and outcome after subarachnoid hemorrhage. *Jama*. 2004; **291**: 866-69.
83 Edlow J. Diagnosing headache in the emergency department: what is more important? Being right, or not being wrong? : Wiley Online Library, 2008; 1257-58.
84 Korja M, Kivisaari R, Rezai Jahromi B, Lehto H. Natural history of ruptured but untreated intracranial aneurysms. *Stroke*. 2017; **48**: 1081-84.
85 Lantigua H, Ortega-Gutierrez S, Schmidt JM, *et al.* Subarachnoid hemorrhage: who dies, and why? *Critical care*. 2015; **19**: 1-10.
86 Connolly Jr ES, Rabinstein AA, Carhuapoma JR, *et al.* Guidelines for the management of aneurysmal subarachnoid hemorrhage: a guideline for healthcare professionals from the American Heart Association/American Stroke Association. *Stroke*. 2012; **43**: 1711-37.
87 Schatlo B, Fung C, Stienen MN, *et al.* Incidence and outcome of aneurysmal subarachnoid hemorrhage: the Swiss Study on Subarachnoid Hemorrhage (Swiss SOS). *Stroke*. 2021; **52**: 344-47.

88 Schuette AJ, Barrow DL. Epidemiology and long-term mortality in subarachnoid hemorrhage. *World Neurosurgery*. 2012; **80**: 264-65.
89 Johnston SC, Selvin S, Gress DR. The burden, trends, and demographics of mortality from subarachnoid hemorrhage. *Neurology*. 1998; **50**: 1413-18.
90 Nicholson P, O'Hare A, Power S, *et al.* Decreasing incidence of subarachnoid hemorrhage. *Journal of NeuroInterventional Surgery*. 2019; **11**: 320-22.
91 Van Gijn J, Kerr RS, Rinkel GJ. Subarachnoid haemorrhage. *The Lancet*. 2007; **369**: 306-18.
92 Eden S, Meurer W, Sanchez B, *et al.* Gender and ethnic differences in subarachnoid hemorrhage. *Neurology*. 2008; **71**: 731-35.
93 Chung AG, Frye JB, Zbesko JC, *et al.* Liquefaction of the brain following stroke shares a similar molecular and morphological profile with atherosclerosis and mediates secondary neurodegeneration in an osteopontin-dependent mechanism. *eneuro*. 2018; **5**.
94 Gualerzi A, Picciolini S, Rodà F, Bedoni M. Extracellular vesicles in regeneration and rehabilitation recovery after stroke. *Biology*. 2021; **10**: 843.
95 Lee T-K, Lu C-Y, Tsai S-T, *et al.* Complete restoration of motor function in acute cerebral stroke treated with allogeneic human umbilical cord blood monocytes: preliminary results of a phase I clinical trial. *Cell Transplantation*. 2021; **30**: 09636897211067447.
96 Liu S, Levine SR, Winn HR. Targeting ischemic penumbra: part I-from pathophysiology to therapeutic strategy. *Journal of experimental stroke & translational medicine*. 2010; **3**: 47.
97 Wang Z-K, Xue L, Wang T, Wang X-J, Su Z-Q. Infiltration of invariant natural killer T cells occur and accelerate brain infarction in permanent ischemic stroke in mice. *Neuroscience letters*. 2016; **633**: 62-68.
98 Slujitoru A-S, Enache A-L, Pintea IL, *et al.* Clinical and morphological correlations in acute ischemic stroke. *Romanian Journal of Morphology and Embryology= Revue Roumaine de Morphologie et Embryologie*. 2012; **53**: 917-26.
99 Jin J. Warning Signs of a Stroke. *JAMA*. 2014; **311**: 1704-04.

100 Birnbaum M, Brock K, Parkinson S, Burton E, Clark R, Hill KD. Rasch analysis of the Burke Lateropulsion Scale (BLS). *Topics in Stroke Rehabilitation*. 2021; **28**: 268-75.
101 Choi T-Y, Ang L, Jun JH, *et al.* Acupuncture and electroacupuncture for stroke: A protocol for overview of systematic review and meta-analysis. *Medicine*. 2022; **101**.
102 Ojaghihaghighi S, Vahdati SS, Mikaeilpour A, Ramouz A. Comparison of neurological clinical manifestation in patients with hemorrhagic and ischemic stroke. *World journal of emergency medicine*. 2017; **8**: 34.
103 Nannoni S, de Groot R, Bell S, Markus HS. Stroke in COVID-19: a systematic review and meta-analysis. *International Journal of Stroke*. 2021; **16**: 137-49.
104 Feigin VL, Roth GA, Naghavi M, *et al.* Global burden of stroke and risk factors in 188 countries, during 1990–2013: a systematic analysis for the Global Burden of Disease Study 2013. *The Lancet Neurology*. 2016; **15**: 913-24.
105 Chiuve SE, Rexrode KM, Spiegelman D, Logroscino G, Manson JE, Rimm EB. Primary prevention of stroke by healthy lifestyle. *Circulation*. 2008; **118**: 947-54.
106 Boehme AK, Esenwa C, Elkind MS. Stroke risk factors, genetics, and prevention. *Circulation research*. 2017; **120**: 472-95.
107 Edzie EKM, Gorleku PN, Dzefi-Tettey K, *et al.* Incidence rate and age of onset of first stroke from CT scan examinations in Cape Coast metropolis. *Heliyon*. 2021; **7**: e06214.
108 Members WG, Roger VL, Go AS, *et al.* Executive summary: heart disease and stroke statistics—2011 update: a report from the American Heart Association. *Circulation*. 2011; **123**: 459-63.
109 Sealy-Jefferson S, Wing JJ, Sánchez BN, *et al.* Age-and ethnic-specific sex differences in stroke risk. *Gender medicine*. 2012; **9**: 121-28.
110 Petrea RE, Beiser AS, Seshadri S, Kelly-Hayes M, Kase CS, Wolf PA. Gender differences in stroke incidence and poststroke disability in the Framingham heart study. *Stroke*. 2009; **40**: 1032-37.
111 Sanchez JM, Jolly SE, Dewland TA, *et al.* Incident strokes among American Indian individuals with atrial

fibrillation. *Journal of the American Heart Association*. 2021; **10**: e019581.
112 Kissela B, Schneider A, Kleindorfer D, *et al.* Stroke in a biracial population: the excess burden of stroke among blacks. *Stroke*. 2004; **35**: 426-31.
113 Collaborators NMSS, Sacco RL, Boden-Albala B, *et al.* Stroke incidence among white, black, and Hispanic residents of an urban community: the Northern Manhattan Stroke Study. *American journal of epidemiology*. 1998; **147**: 259-68.
114 Song S, Liang L, Fonarow GC, *et al.* Comparison of clinical care and in-hospital outcomes of Asian American and white patients with acute ischemic stroke. *JAMA neurology*. 2019; **76**: 430-39.
115 Pourasgari M, Mohamadkhani A. Heritability for stroke: essential for taking family history. *Caspian Journal of Internal Medicine*. 2020; **11**: 237.
116 Whelton PK, Carey RM, Aronow WS, *et al.* 2017 ACC/AHA/AAPA/ABC/ACPM/AGS/APhA/ASH/ASPC/NMA/PCNA guideline for the prevention, detection, evaluation, and management of high blood pressure in adults: a report of the American College of Cardiology/American Heart Association Task Force on Clinical Practice Guidelines. *Journal of the American College of Cardiology*. 2018; **71**: e127-e248.
117 Virani SS, Alonso A, Benjamin EJ, *et al.* Heart disease and stroke statistics—2020 update: a report from the American Heart Association. *Circulation*. 2020; **141**: e139-e596.
118 Weiss J, Freeman M, Low A, Fu R, Kerfoot A, Paynter R. Benefits and Harms of Intensive Blood Pressure Treatment in Adults Aged 60 Years or Older (vol 166, pg 419, 2017). *ANNALS OF INTERNAL MEDICINE*. 2018; **168**: 159-59.
119 O'Conor EC, Wang J, Gibney KD, *et al.* Lowering systolic blood pressure does not increase stroke risk: an analysis of the SPRINT and ACCORD trial data. *Annals of Clinical and Translational Neurology*. 2019; **6**: 144-53.
120 Alloubani A, Saleh A, Abdelhafiz I. Hypertension and diabetes mellitus as a predictive risk factors for stroke.

Diabetes & Metabolic Syndrome: Clinical Research & Reviews. 2018; **12**: 577-84.
121 Psaltopoulou T, Sergentanis TN, Panagiotakos DB, Sergentanis IN, Kosti R, Scarmeas N. Mediterranean diet, stroke, cognitive impairment, and depression: a meta-analysis. *Annals of neurology*. 2013; **74**: 580-91.
122 Chen G-C, Neelakantan N, Martín-Calvo N, *et al.* Adherence to the Mediterranean diet and risk of stroke and stroke subtypes. *European Journal of Epidemiology*. 2019; **34**: 337-49.
123 Spence JD. Nutrition and risk of stroke. *Nutrients*. 2019; **11**: 647.
124 Kleindorfer DO, Towfighi A, Chaturvedi S, *et al.* 2021 guideline for the prevention of stroke in patients with stroke and transient ischemic attack: a guideline from the American Heart Association/American Stroke Association. *Stroke*. 2021; **52**: e364-e467.
125 Trialists CT. The effects of lowering LDL cholesterol with statin therapy in people at low risk of vascular disease: meta-analysis of individual data from 27 randomised trials. *The Lancet*. 2012; **380**: 581-90.
126 Investigators SPbARiCL. High-dose atorvastatin after stroke or transient ischemic attack. *New England Journal of Medicine*. 2006; **355**: 549-59.
127 Isabel C, Calvet D, Mas J-L. Stroke prevention. *La Presse Médicale*. 2016; **45**: e457-e71.
128 Lu Y, Hajifathalian K, Ezzati M, *et al.* Metabolic mediators of the eff ects of body-mass index, overweight, and obesity on coronary heart disease and stroke: a pooled analysis of 97 prospective cohorts with 1.8 million participants. 2014.
129 Suk S-H, Sacco RL, Boden-Albala B, *et al.* Abdominal obesity and risk of ischemic stroke: the Northern Manhattan Stroke Study. *Stroke*. 2003; **34**: 1586-92.
130 Riaz H, Khan MS, Siddiqi TJ, *et al.* Association between obesity and cardiovascular outcomes: a systematic review and meta-analysis of Mendelian randomization studies. *JAMA network open*. 2018; **1**: e183788-e88.
131 Group LAR. Association of the magnitude of weight loss and changes in physical fitness with long-term cardiovascular disease outcomes in overweight or obese

people with type 2 diabetes: a post-hoc analysis of the Look AHEAD randomised clinical trial. *The lancet Diabetes & endocrinology*. 2016; **4**: 913-21.

132 Pan B, Jin X, Jun L, Qiu S, Zheng Q, Pan M. The relationship between smoking and stroke: a meta-analysis. *Medicine*. 2019; **98**.

133 Malek AM, Cushman M, Lackland DT, Howard G, McClure LA. Secondhand smoke exposure and stroke: the reasons for geographic and racial differences in stroke (REGARDS) study. *American journal of preventive medicine*. 2015; **49**: e89-e97.

134 Pirie K, Peto R, Reeves GK, Green J, Beral V. The 21st century hazards of smoking and benefits of stopping: a prospective study of one million women in the UK. *The Lancet*. 2013; **381**: 133-41.

135 Flach C, Muruet W, Wolfe CD, Bhalla A, Douiri A. Risk and secondary prevention of stroke recurrence: a population-base cohort study. *Stroke*. 2020; **51**: 2435-44.

136 Modrego P, Pina M, Mar Fraj M, Llorens N. Type, causes, and prognosis of stroke recurrence in the province of Teruel, Spain. A 5-year analysis. *Neurological Sciences*. 2000; **21**: 355-60.

137 Unnithan AKA, Mehta P. Hemorrhagic stroke. 2020.

138 Sandercock PA, Counsell C, Kane EJ. Anticoagulants for acute ischaemic stroke. *Cochrane Database of Systematic Reviews*. 2015.

139 Lakhan SE, Sapko MT. Blood pressure lowering treatment for preventing stroke recurrence: a systematic review and meta-analysis. *International archives of medicine*. 2009; **2**: 1-8.

140 Arwert HJ, Meesters JJ, Boiten J, Balk F, Wolterbeek R, Vlieland TPV. Poststroke depression: a long-term problem for stroke survivors. *American journal of physical medicine & rehabilitation*. 2018; **97**: 565-71.

141 Towfighi A, Ovbiagele B, El Husseini N, *et al.* Poststroke depression: a scientific statement for healthcare professionals from the American Heart Association/American Stroke Association. *Stroke*. 2017; **48**: e30-e43.

142 Wu Q-e, Zhou A-m, Han Y-p, *et al.* Poststroke depression and risk of recurrent stroke: A meta-analysis of prospective studies. *Medicine*. 2019; **98**.
143 Hosseininezhad M, Sohrabnejad R. Stroke mimics in patients with clinical signs of stroke. *Caspian journal of internal medicine*. 2017; **8**: 213.
144 Roser SM, Bouloux GF. Medical Management and Preoperative Patient Assessment. *Peterson's Principles of Oral and Maxillofacial Surgery*: Springer, 2022; 19-51.
145 Kowalska M, Prendecki M, Kozubski W, Lianeri M, Dorszewska J. Molecular factors in migraine. *Oncotarget*. 2016; **7**: 50708.
146 JE H. Guyton and Hall textbook of medical physiology. *Philadelphia, PA: Saunders Elsevier*. 2011; **107**.
147 Tajti J, Párdutz Á, Vámos E, *et al.* Migraine is a neuronal disease. *Journal of neural transmission*. 2011; **118**: 511-24.
148 Johnson MP, Fernandez F, Colson NJ, Griffiths LR. A pharmacogenomic evaluation of migraine therapy. *Expert opinion on pharmacotherapy*. 2007; **8**: 1821-35.
149 McFaline-Figueroa JR, Lee EQ. Brain tumors. *The American journal of medicine*. 2018; **131**: 874-82.
150 Sabahi M, Hanaei S, Rezaei N. Interdisciplinary Approach in Head and Neck Cancers. Springer, 2022.
151 Rohit K, Tejeswini D. Review on Primary Brain Tumor Diagnosis and Treatment Strategies.
152 Dougherty JM, Carney M, Emmady PD. Vestibular dysfunction. 2020.
153 Gilden DH. Bell's palsy. *New England Journal of Medicine*. 2004; **351**: 1323-31.
154 Carlson DS, Pfadt E. When your patient has acute facial paralysis. *Nursing2021*. 2005; **35**: 54-55.
155 Feghali J, Yang W, Huang J. Updates in chronic subdural hematoma: epidemiology, etiology, pathogenesis, treatment, and outcome. *World neurosurgery*. 2020; **141**: 339-45.
156 Yang W, Huang J. Chronic subdural hematoma: epidemiology and natural history. *Neurosurgery Clinics*. 2017; **28**: 205-10.
157 Panda SP, Soni U. A review of dementia, focusing on the distinct roles of viral protein corona and MMP9 in

dementia: Potential pharmacotherapeutic priorities. *Ageing Research Reviews*. 2022: 101560.
158 Serwer P, Wright ET. A protein assembly hypothesis for population-specific decrease in dementia with time. *Biophysica*. 2021; **1**: 15-21.
159 Control CfD. About Dementia. 2019. (Also available from: https://www.cdc.gov/aging/dementia/index.html, accessed 02/06/2023).
160 H. Buck B, Akhtar N, Alrohimi A, Khan K, Shuaib A. Stroke mimics: incidence, aetiology, clinical features and treatment. *Annals of Medicine*. 2021; **53**: 420-36.
161 Jäger T, Bäzner H, Kliegel M, Szabo K, Hennerici MG. The transience and nature of cognitive impairments in transient global amnesia: a meta-analysis. *Journal of Clinical and Experimental Neuropsychology*. 2009; **31**: 8-19.
162 d Stephen C, Caplan LR. Stroke mimics: Transient focal neurological events. *Stroke in the Older Person*. 2020: 51.
163 Nor AM, Ford GA. Misdiagnosis of stroke. *Expert review of neurotherapeutics*. 2007; **7**: 989-1001.
164 Zhelev Z, Walker G, Henschke N, Fridhandler J, Yip S. Prehospital stroke scales as screening tools for early identification of stroke and transient ischemic attack. *Cochrane Database of Systematic Reviews*. 2019.
165 Rudd M, Buck D, Ford GA, Price CI. A systematic review of stroke recognition instruments in hospital and prehospital settings. *Emergency Medicine Journal*. 2016; **33**: 818-22.
166 Brott T, Adams Jr HP, Olinger CP, *et al.* Measurements of acute cerebral infarction: a clinical examination scale. *Stroke*. 1989; **20**: 864-70.
167 Lyden P, Brott T, Tilley B, *et al.* Improved reliability of the NIH Stroke Scale using video training. NINDS TPA Stroke Study Group. *Stroke*. 1994; **25**: 2220-26.
168 Kwah LK, Diong J. National institutes of health stroke scale (NIHSS). *Journal of physiotherapy*. 2014.
169 Green TL, McNair ND, Hinkle JL, *et al.* Care of the patient with acute ischemic stroke (posthyperacute and prehospital discharge): update to 2009 comprehensive nursing care scientific statement: a scientific statement from the American heart association. *Stroke*. 2021; **52**: e179-e97.

170 Caplan LR. *Caplan's stroke*: Cambridge University Press, 2016.
171 Powers WJ, Rabinstein AA, Ackerson T, *et al.* 2018 guidelines for the early management of patients with acute ischemic stroke: a guideline for healthcare professionals from the American Heart Association/American Stroke Association. *stroke*. 2018; **49**: e46-e99.
172 El-Koussy M, Schroth G, Brekenfeld C, Arnold M. Imaging of acute ischemic stroke. *European neurology*. 2014; **72**: 309-16.
173 Ferrara A. Computed tomography in stroke diagnosis, assessment, and treatment. *Radiologic Technology*. 2020; **91**: 447CT-62CT.
174 Lin MP, Liebeskind DS. Imaging of ischemic stroke. *Continuum: Lifelong Learning in Neurology*. 2016; **22**: 1399.
175 Lansberg MG, Albers GW, Beaulieu C, Marks MP. Comparison of diffusion-weighted MRI and CT in acute stroke. *Neurology*. 2000; **54**: 1557-61.
176 Shafaat O, Sotoudeh H. Stroke imaging. 2019.
177 Li W, Li Y, Qin W, *et al.* Magnetic resonance image (MRI) synthesis from brain computed tomography (CT) images based on deep learning methods for magnetic resonance (MR)-guided radiotherapy. *Quantitative imaging in medicine and surgery*. 2020; **10**: 1223.
178 Frade HC, Wilson SE, Beckwith A, Powers WJ. Comparison of outcomes of ischemic stroke initially imaged with cranial computed tomography alone vs computed tomography plus magnetic resonance imaging. *JAMA Network Open*. 2022; **5**: e2219416-e16.
179 HERSHEY P. Diagnostic Imaging At Rural Hospitals. *Health Affairs*. 2020; **39**: 5.
180 MRI More Sensitive than CT in Diagnosing Stroke. *Emergency Medicine News*. 2007; **29**: 29.
181 Chalela JA, Kidwell CS, Nentwich LM, *et al.* Magnetic resonance imaging and computed tomography in emergency assessment of patients with suspected acute stroke: a prospective comparison. *The Lancet*. 2007; **369**: 293-98.
182 Saver JL. Time is brain—quantified. *Stroke*. 2006; **37**: 263-66.

183 Lakhan SE, Kirchgessner A, Hofer M. Inflammatory mechanisms in ischemic stroke: therapeutic approaches. *Journal of translational medicine*. 2009; **7**: 1-11.
184 Baird AE, Jackson R, Jin W. Tenecteplase for acute ischemic stroke treatment. *Seminars in Neurology*: Thieme Medical Publishers, Inc., 2021; 028-38.
185 Hacke W, Kaste M, Bluhmki E, *et al.* Thrombolysis with alteplase 3 to 4.5 hours after acute ischemic stroke. *New England journal of medicine*. 2008; **359**: 1317-29.
186 dela Peña I, Borlongan C, Shen G, Davis W. Strategies to extend thrombolytic time window for ischemic stroke treatment: an unmet clinical need. *Journal of stroke*. 2017; **19**: 50.
187 Madsen TE, Melluzzo S, Wira CR, *et al.* Minorities, women, and stroke belters left behind in t-PA use despite quality improvement efforts. *Stroke*. 2017; **48**: A116-A16.
188 Henderson SJ, Weitz JI, Kim PY. Fibrinolysis: strategies to enhance the treatment of acute ischemic stroke. *Journal of Thrombosis and Haemostasis*. 2018; **16**: 1932-40.
189 Munich SA, Vakharia K, Levy EI. Overview of mechanical thrombectomy techniques. *Neurosurgery*. 2019; **85**: S60-S67.
190 Mathews S, De Jesus O. Thrombectomy. *StatPearls [Internet]*: StatPearls Publishing, 2021.
191 McCarthy DJ, Diaz A, Sheinberg DL, *et al.* Long-term outcomes of mechanical thrombectomy for stroke: a meta-analysis. *The Scientific World Journal*. 2019; **2019**.
192 Jovin TG, Nogueira RG, Investigators D. Thrombectomy 6 to 24 hours after stroke. *N Engl J Med*. 2018; **378**: 1161-62.
193 De Herdt V, Dumont F, Hénon H, *et al.* Early seizures in intracerebral hemorrhage: incidence, associated factors, and outcome. *Neurology*. 2011; **77**: 1794-800.
194 Hemphill III JC, Greenberg SM, Anderson CS, *et al.* Guidelines for the management of spontaneous intracerebral hemorrhage: a guideline for healthcare professionals from the American Heart Association/American Stroke Association. *Stroke*. 2015; **46**: 2032-60.
195 Park S, Shin IY. The outcomes of suboccipital craniotomy with obtuse-angled partial bone flap comparing

with craniectomy in cerebellar hemorrhage or infarction. *Journal of Korean Skull Base Society*. 2022; **17**: 99-104.
196 Feletti A, Fiorindi A. Hemorrhagic stroke: endoscopic aspiration. *Cerebrovascular Surgery: Controversies, Standards and Advances*: Springer, 2022; 97-119.
197 Richards CL, Malouin F, Nadeau S. Stroke rehabilitation: clinical picture, assessment, and therapeutic challenge. *Progress in brain research*. 2015; **218**: 253-80.
198 Network CS. The quality of stroke care in Canada. *Ottawa: Canadian Stroke Network*. 2011.
199 Heidenreich PA, Trogdon JG, Khavjou OA, *et al.* Forecasting the future of cardiovascular disease in the United States: a policy statement from the American Heart Association. *Circulation*. 2011; **123**: 933-44.
200 Su Y, Yuki M, Otsuki M. Prevalence of stroke-related sarcopenia: A systematic review and meta-analysis. *Journal of Stroke and Cerebrovascular Diseases*. 2020; **29**: 105092.
201 Mohamed JS, Ferrandi PJ, Hector PG, Pitzer CR, Alway SE. Abstract P806: Sirtuin1 Plays a Critical Role in Reversing Skeletal Muscle Atrophy in Cerebral Ischemic Stroke. *Stroke*. 2021; **52**: AP806-AP06.
202 Roshanzamir S. Post stroke rehabilitation. *Galen Medical Journal*. 2016; **5**: 62-65.
203 Stinear CM, Lang CE, Zeiler S, Byblow WD. Advances and challenges in stroke rehabilitation. *The Lancet Neurology*. 2020; **19**: 348-60.
204 Jørgensen HS, Nakayama H, Raaschou HO, Vive-Larsen J, Støier M, Olsen TS. Outcome and time course of recovery in stroke. Part I: Outcome. The Copenhagen Stroke Study. *Archives of physical medicine and rehabilitation*. 1995; **76**: 399-405.
205 Duncan PW, Lai SM, Keighley J. Defining post-stroke recovery: implications for design and interpretation of drug trials. *Neuropharmacology*. 2000; **39**: 835-41.
206 Gadidi V, Katz-Leurer M, Carmeli E, Bornstein NM. Long-term outcome poststroke: predictors of activity limitation and participation restriction. *Archives of physical medicine and rehabilitation*. 2011; **92**: 1802-08.
207 Hendricks HT, Van Limbeek J, Geurts AC, Zwarts MJ. Motor recovery after stroke: a systematic review of the

literature. *Archives of physical medicine and rehabilitation*. 2002; **83**: 1629-37.
208 Health NIo. Post-stroke rehabilitation fact sheet. 2018.
209 Plant S, Tyson SF. A multicentre study of how goal-setting is practised during inpatient stroke rehabilitation. *Clinical rehabilitation*. 2018; **32**: 263-72.
210 Langhorne P, Bernhardt J, Kwakkel G. Stroke rehabilitation. *The Lancet*. 2011; **377**: 1693-702.
211 Crawford L, Maxwell J, Colquhoun H, *et al.* Facilitators and barriers to patient-centred goal-setting in rehabilitation: A scoping review. *Clinical Rehabilitation*. 2022; **36**: 1694-704.
212 Rosewilliam S, Roskell CA, Pandyan A. A systematic review and synthesis of the quantitative and qualitative evidence behind patient-centred goal setting in stroke rehabilitation. *Clinical rehabilitation*. 2011; **25**: 501-14.
213 Brewer L, Horgan F, Hickey A, Williams D. Stroke rehabilitation: recent advances and future therapies. *QJM: An International Journal of Medicine*. 2013; **106**: 11-25.
214 Trialists'Collaboration SU. Organised inpatient (stroke unit) care for stroke. *Cochrane database syst rev*. 2013; **9**.
215 Clarke DJ. The role of multidisciplinary team care in stroke rehabilitation. *Progress in Neurology and Psychiatry*. 2013; **17**: 5-8.
216 Welch JF, Sutor T, Vose AK, Perim RR, Fox EJ, Mitchell GS. Synergy between acute intermittent hypoxia and task-specific training. *Exercise and sport sciences reviews*. 2020; **48**: 125.
217 Boyd LA, Vidoni ED, Wessel BD. Motor learning after stroke: is skill acquisition a prerequisite for contralesional neuroplastic change? *Neuroscience letters*. 2010; **482**: 21-25.
218 Committee ESOE, Committee EW. Guidelines for management of ischaemic stroke and transient ischaemic attack 2008. *Cerebrovascular diseases*. 2008; **25**: 457-507.
219 Stephan KM, Pérennou D. Mobility After Stroke: Relearning to Walk. *Clinical Pathways in Stroke Rehabilitation: Evidence-based Clinical Practice Recommendations*. 2021: 123-47.

220 De Wit L, Putman K, Dejaeger E, *et al*. Use of time by stroke patients: a comparison of four European rehabilitation centers. *Stroke*. 2005; **36**: 1977-83.
221 Connell LA, Klassen TK, Janssen J, Thetford C, Eng JJ. Delivering intensive rehabilitation in stroke: factors influencing implementation. *Physical therapy*. 2018; **98**: 243-50.
222 Bernhardt J, Hayward KS, Kwakkel G, *et al*. Agreed definitions and a shared vision for new standards in stroke recovery research: the stroke recovery and rehabilitation roundtable taskforce. *Neurorehabilitation and neural repair*. 2017; **31**: 793-99.
223 Lai C-L, Tsai M-M, Luo J-Y, Liao W-C, Hsu P-S, Chen H-Y. Post-acute care for stroke–a retrospective cohort study in Taiwan. *Patient preference and adherence*. 2017: 1309-15.
224 Wood-Dauphinee S, Williams JI. Reintegration to normal living as a proxy to quality of life. *Journal of chronic diseases*. 1987; **40**: 491-99.
225 Obembe A, Mapayi B, Johnson O, Agunbiade T, Emechete A. Community reintegration in stroke survivors: Relationship with motor function and depression. *Hong Kong Physiotherapy Journal*. 2013; **31**: 69-74.
226 Ilett PA, Brock KA, Graven CJ, Cotton SM. Selecting patients for rehabilitation after acute stroke: are there variations in practice? *Archives of physical medicine and rehabilitation*. 2010; **91**: 788-93.
227 Buntin MB, Garten AD, Paddock S, Saliba D, Totten M, Escarce JJ. How much is postacute care use affected by its availability? *Health services research*. 2005; **40**: 413-34.
228 Medicare Cf, Services M. Medicare and Medicaid programs; revisions to requirements for discharge planning for hospitals, critical access hospitals, and home health agencies. *Federal Register*. 2019; **84**: 51836-84.
229 Miller EL, Murray L, Richards L, *et al*. Comprehensive overview of nursing and interdisciplinary rehabilitation care of the stroke patient: a scientific statement from the American Heart Association. *Stroke*. 2010; **41**: 2402-48.
230 Belagaje SR. Stroke rehabilitation. *CONTINUUM: Lifelong Learning in Neurology*. 2017; **23**: 238-53.

231 Winstein CJ, Stein J, Arena R, *et al.* Guidelines for adult stroke rehabilitation and recovery: a guideline for healthcare professionals from the American Heart Association/American Stroke Association. *Stroke.* 2016; **47**: e98-e169.
232 Simmonds KP, Burke J, Kozlowski AJ, Andary M, Luo Z, Reeves MJ. Rationale for a clinical trial that compares acute stroke rehabilitation at inpatient rehabilitation facilities to skilled nursing facilities: Challenges and opportunities. *Archives of Physical Medicine and Rehabilitation.* 2022; **103**: 1213-21.
233 Dąbrowski J, Czajka A, Zielińska-Turek J, *et al.* Brain functional reserve in the context of neuroplasticity after stroke. *Neural Plasticity.* 2019.
234 Burke SN, Barnes CA. Neural plasticity in the ageing brain. *Nature reviews neuroscience.* 2006; **7**: 30-40.
235 Mateos-Aparicio P, Rodríguez-Moreno A. The impact of studying brain plasticity. *Frontiers in cellular neuroscience.* 2019; **13**: 66.
236 Pascual-Leone A, Amedi A, Fregni F, Merabet LB. The plastic human brain cortex. *Annu Rev Neurosci.* 2005; **28**: 377-401.
237 Johansson B. Current trends in stroke rehabilitation. A review with focus on brain plasticity. *Acta Neurologica Scandinavica.* 2011; **123**: 147-59.
238 Ekusheva E, Damulin I. Post-stroke rehabilitation: importance of neuroplasticity and sensorimotor integration processes. *Neuroscience and Behavioral Physiology.* 2015; **45**: 594-99.
239 Berlucchi G, Buchtel HA. Neuronal plasticity: historical roots and evolution of meaning. *Experimental brain research.* 2009; **192**: 307-19.
240 Veerbeek JM, van Wegen E, van Peppen R, *et al.* What is the evidence for physical therapy poststroke? A systematic review and meta-analysis. *PloS one.* 2014; **9**: e87987.
241 Kwakkel G, Veerbeek JM, van Wegen EE, Wolf SL. Constraint-induced movement therapy after stroke. *The Lancet Neurology.* 2015; **14**: 224-34.

242 Tyson SF, Hanley M, Chillala J, Selley A, Tallis RC. Balance disability after stroke. *Physical therapy*. 2006; **86**: 30-38.
243 Michael KM, Allen JK, Macko RF. Reduced ambulatory activity after stroke: the role of balance, gait, and cardiovascular fitness. *Archives of physical medicine and rehabilitation*. 2005; **86**: 1552-56.
244 Macias JD, Massingale S, Gerkin RD. Efficacy of vestibular rehabilitation therapy in reducing falls. *Otolaryngology—Head and Neck Surgery*. 2005; **133**: 323-25.
245 Rensink M, Schuurmans M, Lindeman E, Hafsteinsdottir T. Task-oriented training in rehabilitation after stroke: systematic review. *Journal of advanced nursing*. 2009; **65**: 737-54.
246 Takeuchi N, Izumi S-I. Rehabilitation with poststroke motor recovery: a review with a focus on neural plasticity. *Stroke research and treatment*. 2013; **2013**.
247 McCain KJ, Pollo FE, Baum BS, Coleman SC, Baker S, Smith PS. Locomotor treadmill training with partial body-weight support before overground gait in adults with acute stroke: a pilot study. *Archives of physical medicine and rehabilitation*. 2008; **89**: 684-91.
248 Maier M, Ballester BR, Leiva Bañuelos N, Duarte Oller E, Verschure PF. Adaptive conjunctive cognitive training (ACCT) in virtual reality for chronic stroke patients: a randomized controlled pilot trial. *Journal of neuroengineering and rehabilitation*. 2020; **17**: 1-20.
249 Farokhi-Sisakht F, Farhoudi M, Sadigh-Eteghad S, Mahmoudi J, Mohaddes G. Cognitive rehabilitation improves ischemic stroke-induced cognitive impairment: role of growth factors. *Journal of Stroke and Cerebrovascular Diseases*. 2019; **28**: 104299.
250 Cattelani R, Zettin M, Zoccolotti P. Rehabilitation treatments for adults with behavioral and psychosocial disorders following acquired brain injury: A systematic review. *Neuropsychology review*. 2010; **20**: 52-85.
251 Skidmore ER, Whyte EM, Holm MB, *et al.* Cognitive and affective predictors of rehabilitation participation after stroke. *Archives of physical medicine and rehabilitation*. 2010; **91**: 203-07.

252 Loetscher T, Potter KJ, Wong D, das Nair R. Cognitive rehabilitation for attention deficits following stroke. *Cochrane Database of Systematic Reviews*. 2019.

253 Bowen A, Patchick E. Cognitive rehabilitation and recovery after stroke. *The Behavioral Consequences of Stroke*. 2014: 315-39.

254 Parsons TD. Neuropsychological Rehabilitation 3.0: State of the Science. *Clinical Neuropsychology and Technology: What's New and How We Can Use It*. 2016: 113-32.

255 Solana J, Cáceres C, García-Molina A, *et al*. Improving brain injury cognitive rehabilitation by personalized telerehabilitation services: Guttmann neuropersonal trainer. *IEEE journal of biomedical and health informatics*. 2014; **19**: 124-31.

256 Bailey RR. Lifestyle modification for secondary stroke prevention. *American journal of lifestyle medicine*. 2018; **12**: 140-47.

257 Tang EYH, Robinson L, Price C. Stroke: time to address cognition. British Journal of General Practice, 2021; 104-05.

258 A randomised b, trial of clopidogrel versus aspirin in patients at risk of ischaemic events. CAPRIE steering committee. *Lancet*. 1996; **348**: 1329-39.

259 Johnston SC, Easton JD, Farrant M, *et al*. Clopidogrel and aspirin in acute ischemic stroke and high-risk TIA. *New England Journal of Medicine*. 2018; **379**: 215-25.

260 Barnett HJ, Taylor DW, Eliasziw M, *et al*. Benefit of carotid endarterectomy in patients with symptomatic moderate or severe stenosis. *New England Journal of Medicine*. 1998; **339**: 1415-25.

261 Manns PJ, Dunstan DW, Owen N, Healy GN. Addressing the nonexercise part of the activity continuum: a more realistic and achievable approach to activity programming for adults with mobility disability? *Physical therapy*. 2012; **92**: 614-25.

262 Ivey FM, Macko R, Ryan A, Hafer-Macko C. Cardiovascular health and fitness after stroke. *Topics in stroke rehabilitation*. 2005; **12**: 1-16.

263 Ivey FM, Hafer-Macko CE, Macko RF. Exercise training for cardiometabolic adaptation after stroke. *Journal of cardiopulmonary rehabilitation and prevention*. 2008; **28**: 2-11.

264 Gardiner PA, Eakin EG, Healy GN, Owen N. Feasibility of reducing older adults' sedentary time. *American journal of preventive medicine*. 2011; **41**: 174-77.
265 English C, MacDonald-Wicks L, Patterson A, Attia J, Hankey GJ. The role of diet in secondary stroke prevention. *The Lancet Neurology*. 2021; **20**: 150-60.
266 Chen J, Li S, Zheng K, *et al.* Impact of smoking status on stroke recurrence. *Journal of the American Heart Association*. 2019; **8**: e011696.
267 Yu-Jie W, Hui-Liang L, Bing L, Lu Z, Zhi-Geng J. Impact of smoking and smoking cessation on arterial stiffness in healthy participants. *Angiology*. 2013; **64**: 273-80.
268 Zawawi N, Aziz N, Fisher R, Ahmad K, Walker MF. The unmet needs of stroke survivors and stroke caregivers: a systematic narrative review. *Journal of Stroke and Cerebrovascular Diseases*. 2020; **29**: 104875.
269 Rigby H, Gubitz G, Phillips S. A systematic review of caregiver burden following stroke. *International Journal of Stroke*. 2009; **4**: 285-92.
270 Menon B, Salini P, Habeeba K, Conjeevaram J, Munisusmitha K. Female caregivers and stroke severity determines caregiver stress in stroke patients. *Annals of Indian Academy of Neurology*. 2017; **20**: 418.
271 Kokorelias KM, Lu FK, Santos JR, Xu Y, Leung R, Cameron JI. "Caregiving is a full-time job" impacting stroke caregivers' health and well-being: A qualitative meta-synthesis. *Health & social care in the community*. 2020; **28**: 325-40.
272 Smith LN, Lawrence M, Kerr SM, Langhorne P, Lees KR. Informal carers' experience of caring for stroke survivors. *Journal of advanced nursing*. 2004; **46**: 235-44.
273 Coombs UE. Spousal caregiving for stroke survivors. *Journal of Neuroscience Nursing*. 2007; **39**: 112-19.
274 Oliva-Moreno J, Peña-Longobardo LM, Mar J, *et al.* Determinants of informal care, burden, and risk of burnout in caregivers of stroke survivors: the CONOCES study. *Stroke*. 2018; **49**: 140-46.
275 Beydoun J, Nasrallah L, Sabrah T, Caboral-Stevens M. Towards a definition of caregiver fatigue: a concept analysis. *Advances in Nursing Science*. 2019; **42**: 297-306.

276 Hartke R, King R. The effectiveness of a telephone support group for stroke caregivers. *Journal of Rehabilitation Research and Development*. 1997; **34**: 124.
277 Olai L, Borgquist L, Svärdsudd K. Life situations and the care burden for stroke patients and their informal caregivers in a prospective cohort study. *Upsala journal of medical sciences*. 2015; **120**: 290-98.
278 Silva-Smith AL. Restructuring life: Preparing for and beginning a new caregiving role. *Journal of family nursing*. 2007; **13**: 99-116.
279 Cecil R, Thompson K, Parahoo K, McCaughan E. Towards an understanding of the lives of families affected by stroke: a qualitative study of home carers. *Journal of Advanced Nursing*. 2013; **69**: 1761-70.
280 Thompson T, Pierce L, Steiner V, Govoni A, Hicks B, Friedemann M. What happened to normal? Learning the role of caregiver. *Online Journal of Nursing Informatics*. 2004; **8**.
281 Barbic SP, Mayo NE, White CL, Bartlett SJ. Emotional vitality in family caregivers: content validation of a theoretical framework. *Quality of Life Research*. 2014; **23**: 2865-72.
282 Buschenfeld K, Morris R, Lockwood S. The experience of partners of young stroke survivors. *Disability and rehabilitation*. 2009; **31**: 1643-51.
283 Kum C, Miller EL, Jones H, Kean EB, Kreitzer N, Bakas T. Theoretically based factors affecting stroke family caregiver health: An integrative review. *Western Journal of Nursing Research*. 2022; **44**: 338-51.
284 Prevention CfDCa. Caregiving for family and friends—a public health issue. 2019.
285 Li T-C, Lee Y-D, Lin C-C, Amidon RL. Quality of life of primary caregivers of elderly with cerebrovascular disease or diabetes hospitalized for acute care: assessment of well-being and functioning using the SF-36 health questionnaire. *Quality of Life Research*. 2004; **13**: 1081-88.
286 Ostwald SK, Bernal MP, Cron SG, Godwin KM. Stress experienced by stroke survivors and spousal caregivers during the first year after discharge from inpatient rehabilitation. *Topics in stroke rehabilitation*. 2009; **16**: 93-104.

287 Ilse IB, Feys H, De Wit L, Putman K, De Weerdt W. Stroke caregivers' strain: prevalence and determinants in the first six months after stroke. *Disability and Rehabilitation*. 2008; **30**: 523-30.
288 King RB, Ainsworth CR, Ronen M, Hartke RJ. Stroke caregivers: pressing problems reported during the first months of caregiving. *Journal of Neuroscience Nursing*. 2010; **42**: 302-11.
289 Haley WE, Allen JY, Grant JS, Clay OJ, Perkins M, Roth DL. Problems and benefits reported by stroke family caregivers: results from a prospective epidemiological study. *Stroke*. 2009; **40**: 2129-33.
290 Tooth L, Mckenna K, Barnett A, Prescott C, Murphy S. Caregiver burden, time spent caring and health status in the first 12 months following stroke. *Brain Injury*. 2005; **19**: 963-74.
291 Anderson CS, Linto J, Stewart-Wynne EG. A population-based assessment of the impact and burden of caregiving for long-term stroke survivors. *Stroke*. 1995; **26**: 843-49.
292 Reimer WSo, De Haan R, Rijnders P, Limburg M, Van Den Bos G. The burden of caregiving in partners of long-term stroke survivors. *Stroke*. 1998; **29**: 1605-11.
293 Han B, Haley WE. Family caregiving for patients with stroke: review and analysis. *Stroke*. 1999; **30**: 1478-85.
294 Archbold PG, Stewart BJ, Greenlick MR, Harvath T. Mutuality and preparedness as predictors of caregiver role strain. *Research in nursing & health*. 1990; **13**: 375-84.
295 Pierce LL, Steiner V, Govoni AL, Hicks B, Thompson TLC, Friedemann M-L. Caregivers dealing with stroke pull together and feel connected. *Journal of Neuroscience Nursing*. 2004; **36**: 32-39.
296 Bulley C, Shiels J, Wilkie K, Salisbury L. Carer experiences of life after stroke–a qualitative analysis. *Disability and rehabilitation*. 2010; **32**: 1406-13.
297 Kitzmüller G, Häggström T, Asplund K, Gilje FL. The existential meaning of couples' long-term experience of living with stroke. *Illness, Crisis & Loss*. 2012; **20**: 339-62.
298 Ablewhite J, Nouri F, Whisker A, *et al*. How do stroke survivors and their caregivers manage post-stroke fatigue? A qualitative study. *Clinical Rehabilitation*. 2022; **36**: 1400-10.

299 King RB, Raad JH, Flaherty J, Hartke RJ. Stroke Caregiver Depression: Qualitative Comparison of Treatment Responders and Nonresponders at 1 Year. *Journal of Cardiovascular Nursing*. 2022; **37**: 581-88.
300 Camak DJ. Addressing the burden of stroke caregivers: a literature review. *Journal of clinical nursing*. 2015; **24**: 2376-82.
301 Cameron JI, Cheung AM, Streiner DL, Coyte PC, Stewart DE. Stroke survivor depressive symptoms are associated with family caregiver depression during the first 2 years poststroke. *Stroke*. 2011; **42**: 302-06.
302 Panzeri A, Rossi Ferrario S, Vidotto G. Interventions for psychological health of stroke caregivers: a systematic review. *Frontiers in psychology*. 2019; **10**: 2045.
303 Wan-Fei K, Hassan STS, Sann LM, Ismail SIF, Raman RA, Ibrahim F. Depression, anxiety and quality of life in stroke survivors and their family caregivers: A pilot study using an actor/partner interdependence model. *Electronic physician*. 2017; **9**: 4924.
304 Bastawrous M, Gignac MA, Kapral MK, Cameron JI. Adult daughters providing post-stroke care to a parent: a qualitative study of the impact that role overload has on lifestyle, participation and family relationships. *Clinical rehabilitation*. 2015; **29**: 592-600.
305 Sambasivam R, Liu J, Vaingankar JA, *et al.* The hidden patient: chronic physical morbidity, psychological distress, and quality of life in caregivers of older adults. *Psychogeriatrics*. 2019; **19**: 65-72.
306 Lutz BJ, Ellen Young M, Cox KJ, Martz C, Rae Creasy K. The crisis of stroke: experiences of patients and their family caregivers. *Topics in stroke rehabilitation*. 2011; **18**: 786-97.
307 Pucciarelli G, Lyons KS, Petrizzo A, *et al.* Protective role of caregiver preparedness on the relationship between depression and quality of life in stroke dyads. *Stroke*. 2022; **53**: 145-53.
308 Petruzzo A, Biagioli V, Durante A, *et al.* Influence of preparedness on anxiety, depression, and quality of life in caregivers of heart failure patients: testing a model of path analysis. *Patient Education and Counseling*. 2019; **102**: 1021-28.

309 Henriksson A, Årestedt K. Exploring factors and caregiver outcomes associated with feelings of preparedness for caregiving in family caregivers in palliative care: a correlational, cross-sectional study. *Palliative medicine*. 2013; **27**: 639-46.
310 Creasy KR, Lutz BJ, Young ME, Ford A, Martz C. The impact of interactions with providers on stroke caregivers' needs. *Rehabilitation Nursing*. 2013; **38**: 88-98.
311 Mackenzie A, Greenwood N. Positive experiences of caregiving in stroke: a systematic review. *Disability and rehabilitation*. 2012; **34**: 1413-22.
312 Ostwald SK, Godwin KM, Cron SG, Kelley CP, Hersch G, Davis S. Home-based psychoeducational and mailed information programs for stroke-caregiving dyads post-discharge: a randomized trial. *Disability and Rehabilitation*. 2014; **36**: 55-62.

Resources

The following websites provide quality information for stroke survivors and their families/caretakers:

American Stroke Association:

- https://www.stroke.org/en/

American Stroke Foundation:

- https://americanstroke.org/

Centers for Disease Control and Prevention

- https://www.cdc.gov/stroke/about.htm

National Institutes of Health

- https://www.stroke.nih.gov/resources/

Stroke Recovery Foundation:

- https://strokerecoveryfoundation.org/

Stroke Support Association:

- https://strokesupportassoc.org/

The Stroke Network:

- http://www.strokenetwork.org/

World Stroke Organization

- https://www.world-stroke.org/

Note: Many countries have their own stroke websites and resources. If you are reading this from outside the United States, be sure to check for available resources that are specific to your country of residence.

Let others know!

If you found this book informative, *please take the time and post a review online*! Reviews help get exposure for the book and thereby improve the chances that others will be able to benefit from the material as well.

Image Credits

Figure 1.1: Noiel/Shutterstock.com

Figure 1.2: MattLphotography/Shutterstock.com

Figure 1.3: Hank Grebe/Shutterstock.com

Figure 1.4: grayjay/Shutterstock.com

Figure 1.5: MattLphotography/Shutterstock.com

Figure 2.1: Inspiring/Shutterstock.com

Figure 2.2: Jeniffer Fontan/Shutterstock.com

Figure 5.1: Samuel Micut/Shutterstock.com

Figure 5.2: toysf400/Shutterstock.com

Figure 8.1: Svitlana Hulko/Shutterstock.com

Front Cover: Viktoriya/Shutterstock.com

Back Cover: SciePro/Shutterstock.com

About the Author

Mark is a small-town Kansas native who now lives in a suburb of Houston with his wife and two young daughters. His background is in the area of sports medicine, obtaining his bachelor's degree from Wichita State and his master's degree from the University of Nevada, Las Vegas. After working clinically as an athletic trainer for eight years, Mark returned to graduate school where he received his doctorate in Kinesiology from the University of Houston, followed by a postdoctoral assistantship in Molecular Physiology and Biophysics at Baylor College of Medicine in Houston, TX. He has been employed as a college professor at the University of Houston since 2013, eventually achieving the rank of clinical associate professor.

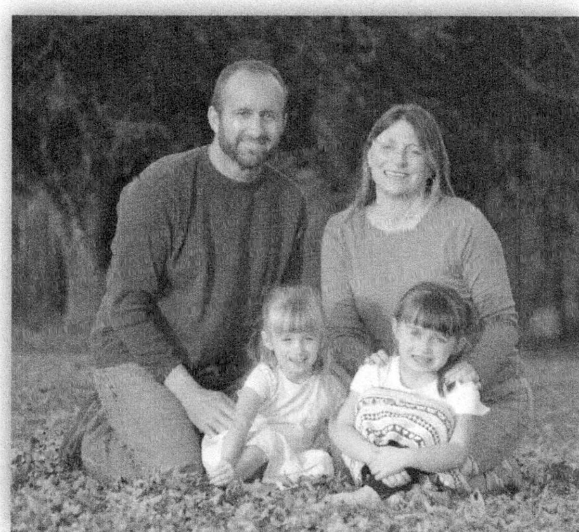

Made in the USA
Monee, IL
13 September 2026

62981967R00134